MW01101110

Shanghai Key Books

上海市重点图书

An English-Chinese Guide to Clinical Treatment of Common Diseases

（英汉对照）常见病临证要览

Typical TCM Therapy for Primary Hypertension

高血压病的中医特色疗法

Compiled by Sa Ronggui　Li qiyi

洒荣桂　李七一　编著

Translated by Huang Yuezhong　Hu Kewu

Wei Min　Qin Baichang

黄月中　胡克武　魏敏　覃百长　翻译

Revised by Ou Ming

欧明　审阅

Shanghai University of Traditional
Chinese Medicine Press

上海中医药大学出版社

图书在版编目（CIP）数据

高血压病的中医特色疗法 / 洒荣桂，李七一编著；黄
月中等译 . —上海：上海中医药大学出版社，2004.7
（（英汉对照）常见病临证要览）
ISBN 7－81010－795－X

Ⅰ.高... Ⅱ.①洒... ②李... ③黄...
Ⅲ.高血压—中医治疗法—英、汉 Ⅳ. R259.441

中国版本图书馆 CIP 数据核字（2004）第 042202号

高血压病的中医特色疗法

洒荣桂 李七一 编著

上海中医药大学出版社出版发行 (http://www.tcmonline.com.cn)

（上海浦东新区蔡伦路 1200 号 邮政编码 201203）

新华书店上海发行所经销 南京展望文化发展有限公司排版 上海市印刷七厂一分厂印刷
开本 850mm × 1168mm 1/32 印张 8.625 字数 173 千字 印数 1－3100 册
版次 2004 年 7 月第 1 版 印次 2004 年 7 月第 1 次印刷

ISBN 7－81010－795－X/R・757 定价：23.00 元
（本书如有印刷、装订问题，请寄回本社出版科，或电话 021－51322545 联系）

Compilation Board of the Guide

《(英汉对照)常见病临证要览》
编纂委员会

主　任　谢建群　吴勉华
副主任　汪　悦　丁年青
主　编　吴勉华　汪　悦
主　译　谢建群
副主编　黄桂成　王　旭
副主译　丁年青　黄国琪

编　委（按姓氏笔画为序）

田开宇	冯　丽	孙玉明	朱玉琴
朱忠宝	乐毅敏	成肇智	李七一
吴　敏	吴承玉	汪腊萍	张　琴
张传儒	沈卫星	杨亚平	杨智军
周　鲁	周　愉	周学平	郑林赟
郑耀玶	胡克武	酒荣桂	赵和庆
唐国顺	顾学兰	徐　瑶	徐小燕
陶锦文	黄月中	覃百长	薛博瑜
魏　敏			

出版人　朱邦贤

中文责任编辑（按姓氏笔画为序）

马胜英	王玲琍	王德良	何倩倩
沈春晖	单宝枝	姜水印	秦葆平
钱静庄	葛德宏		

英文责任编辑　单宝枝　姜水印　肖元春
英文特邀编辑　李照国
美术编辑　王　磊
技术编辑　徐国民

Foreword

Traditional Chinese Medicine (TCM), a great treasure of world medical science, has the history of thousands of years. It has obtained remarkable attraction and reputation in the global medical society with its new image of "nature, security, and effectiveness". More and more people over the world accept the TCM. It is our unshirkable duty, as the descendents of the Chinese doctors, to make TCM in progress so as to benefit the health of human beings.

We compiled the series of "An English-Chinese Guide to Clinical Treatment of Common Diseases" in order to assist foreign students to have a better study of clinical knowledge of TCM. The series also meet the need of Chinese doctors when they spread TCM for foreign practitioners. The series are scientifically-organized reference books which could generally reflect the updated development of clinic in TCM.

The series were written and compiled by medical professionals and English experts from 7 TCM universities or colleges including Nanjing University of TCM,

Shanghai University of TCM, Guangzhou University of TCM, etc.. The faculty from Nanjing University of TCM compiled the Chinese part. Shanghai University of TCM with other colleges and universities were responsible for the translation. The proposal was drafted in 1998. After 5-year continuous adaptation, the whole series were finally completed in 2003.

The first series include ten books. They cover ten commonly-encountered diseases of viral hepatitis, primary glomerulonephritis, chronic gastritis, lung cancer, bronchial asthma, diabetes, primary hypertension, rheumatoid arthritis, cervical spondylosis, and cholelithiasis and their special treatment in traditional Chinese medicine. Each book consists of three parts. Part one discusses the major points in diagnosis and pathogenesis and pathology of the disease. Part two focuses on the typical therapy in TCM. It covers internal therapy, external therapy, acupuncture and moxibustion, Tuina (Chinese massage), physiotherapy, dietetic therapy, mental therapy, and regimen. Part three illustrates the academic experience of 3 – 4 celebrated doctors and the effective cases that they treated.

Wu Mianhua, Wang Yue, Huang Guicheng, Wang Xu and over ten professionals from Nanjing University of TCM have made great contribution. Ding Nianqing,

Huang Guoqi, Zheng Linyun from Shanghai University of TCM, Tao Jinwen from Nanjing University of TCM, Huang Yuezhong from Guangzhou University of TCM, Tian Kaiyu from Henan College of TCM, Le Yimin from Jiangxi College of TCM, Cheng Zhaozhi from Hubei College of TCM, and Tang Guoshun from Shanghai Information Institute of TCM have finished the translation through their diligent work. Professor Ou Ming from Guangzhou University of TCM, Professor Li Zhaoguo from Shanghai University of TCM and Professor Zhu Zhongbao from Henan College of TCM spent their valuable time on the proofreading and adaptation. Acknowledgement is also given to the leaders and editors from Shanghai University of TCM Press for their great support in publishing the series.

All the diseases selected in the series are frequently encountered in the clinic. The description is brief and to the point. The translation is accurate and standard. But it is not easy to precisely translate the theoretical and clinic terminology of TCM into English. Although all the members have made their great efforts, the limitation of the knowledge and different style in composition and translation will still leave the errors and mistakes. Comments and suggestions from colleagues at home and abroad are really appreciated, so that we will make improvement in the revised edition in future.

Xie Jianqun

Shanghai University of Traditional Chinese Medicine

December, 2003

序　言

数千年中华文化历史积淀铸就的中国医药学是世界医学的瑰宝,今天她正以"绿色"、"安全"、"有效"的崭新面貌,赢得了国际医学界的赞誉,也日益为世界上越来越多的国家和人民所接受。将中国传统医学进一步发扬光大,使之造福于全人类的健康,这是我辈岐黄传人义不容辞的职责。

为了使海外留学生能更好地学习中医的临床技能,也为了适应中国临床医师对外传播中医药学的需要,我们组织编写了这套《(英汉对照)常见病临证要览》,旨在提供一套科学规范、能全面反映中医临床诊疗实践与发展的对外交流的教学参考丛书。

本书由南京中医药大学、上海中医药大学、广州中医药大学等7所中医院校有关临床专家和英语教授合作编撰。其中,南京中医药大学负责中医临床等方面内容的编审,上海中医药大学汇合其他各院校负责英语编译。全书的编写大纲草拟于1998年,期间历经反复斟酌、修改,历时五载,终于2003年底基本定稿,可以与中医界同仁和广大读者见面了。

本丛书首先推出10册,每册分上、中、下三篇,分别介绍病毒性肝炎、原发性肾小球肾炎、慢性胃炎、肺癌、支气管哮喘、糖尿病、高血压病、类风湿关节炎、颈椎病及胆石症等临床常见病的中医特色疗法。上篇为总论,概述各病种的诊断要点、病因病机;中篇专论中医对该病症的临床特色疗法,包括内治、外治、针灸、推拿、体疗、食疗、情志疗法、摄生调护等;下篇介绍了3～4位著名老中医的学术经验与医案。

南京中医药大学的吴勉华、汪悦、黄桂成、王旭等10多位专家为本书中文稿的编审付出了很多心血,上海中医药大学的丁年青、黄国琪、郑林赟,南京中医药大学的陶锦文,广州中医药大学的黄月中,河南中医学院的田开宇,江西中医学院的乐毅敏,湖北中医学院的成肇智,以及上海中医药情报研究所的唐国顺等专家为本书的译文尽心尽力;广州中医药大学欧明教授、上海中医药大学李照国教授、河南中医学院朱忠宝教授也为本书译文的润色修饰耗费了很多宝贵的时间,上海中医药大学出版社领导和编辑部的同志们为本书的出版倾注热情,大力支持,在此谨致深深的谢意。

在编写过程中,作者力求做到所选病种常见、多发,文字简明扼要,译文准确规范。然而,要把中医理论及其临床术语翻译为英语,并能准确表述其内涵,难度可想而知。尽管我们作了极大努力,囿于作者的学识,再加上撰写者行文风格的差异,粗疏之处在所难免,诚望海内外同道不吝指教,以便在今后修订时能进一步得以提高和改进。

谢建群
2003 年 12 月
于上海中医药大学

高血压病的中医特色疗法

Preface

Primary hypertension is a kind of cardiovascular disease seriously threatening people's health. For a long period of time, rich experience has been acquired in the prevention and treatment of primary hypertension in traditional Chinese medicine (TCM). During the last 20 years, with the adoption of modern research, there has been a deeper understanding of primary hypertension and there appear more effective treatments for primary hypertension in TCM. This is actually a collection of distinctive TCM therapies, which may contribute to the prevention, treatment and control of primary hypertension.

There are three parts in this book, which, from the viewpoint of TCM, discusses primary hypertension in great detail in various aspects, including etiology, pathogenesis, syndrome differentiation, treatment and prescription, simple prescription and experiential prescription, Chinese patent medicine, as well as application method, fumigation and washing therapy, medicinal pillow, acupuncture and moxibustion, massage, dietotherapy and life-cultivation therapy. In addition, the book introduces some famous senior practitioners' unique understanding of primary hypertension, their personal experience and effective treatments, rich in content and useful in clinical practice.

If readers should come across any mistakes and shortcomings of the book, they are cordially invited to point them out.

Sa Ronggui Li qiyi
December 2003

前　言

　　高血压病是一种严重危害人类身体健康的心血管疾病。中医防治该病历史悠久,积累了丰富的经验。近 20 年来,由于融会、结合现代医学科学的研究成果,使中医对高血压病的认识更加深入、治法不断扩充、疗效逐渐提高。本书力图总结这些成就,突出中医特色优势,以期为高血压病的防治作出一点贡献。

　　全书共分上、中、下三篇,对高血压病的中医病因病机、辨证分型、治法方药、单方验方、中成药,以及敷贴法、薰洗法、药枕、针灸、推拿,乃至食疗、摄生调护,均作了详细的论述与介绍。本书还收集了部分名老中医对本病独特的认识、体会和治法,内容丰富,实用性强。

　　由于编者水平有限,书中有不足之处,尚祈读者指正。

洒荣桂　李七一
2003 年 12 月

高血压病的中医特色疗法

3

Contents

Part One   General Introduction

Chapter One   A Brief Account ························· 2

Chapter Two   Diagnostic Essentials ····················· 4

Chapter Three   Understanding of Primary
Hypertension in TCM ··············· 12

Part Two   Distinctive Treatment

Chapter One   Treatment of Primary
Hypertension ························· 20

Section One   Internal Treatment ················ 20

Section Two   External Therapy ··················· 40

Section Three   Acupuncture-moxibustion
Therapy ························· 44

Section Four   Massage Therapy ····················· 50

Section Five   Physical Exercise Therapy ········· 52

Section Six   Mental Therapy ······················ 56

Section Seven   Dietotherapy ····················· 58

Chapter Two   Treatment for Senile Primary
Hypertension ························· 74

Typical TCM Therapy for Primary Hypertension

Section One   Six "Dos" ································ 82

Section Two   Thirteen "Don'ts" ···················· 84

Chapter Three   Treatment for Chief Manifestations
                 of Primary Hypertension ············ 90

Section One   Headache ······························· 90

Section Two   Dizziness ······························· 92

Section Three   Palpitation ···························· 96

Section Four   Numbness of Extremities ········· 98

Chapter Four   Treatment for Complications of
                Primary Hypertension ·············· 102

Section One   Hypertensive Encephalopathy ······ 102

Section Two   Hypertensive Crisis ·············· 110

Chapter Five   Regimen for Primary Hypertension

                ································ 116

Section One   Body Weight Reduction ············ 116

Section Two   Limitation of Salt Intake ········ 118

Section Three   Abstention from Smoking and
                 Limitation of Alcohol Intake

                 ······························ 118

Section Four   Lifestyle Modification ············ 120

**Part Three   Experience of Famous
Senior TCM Doctors**

Chapter One   Zhou Zhongying's Experience ······ 122

Section One   Understanding of Etiology and

Contents

Pathogenesis ·························· 122

Section Two   Diagnostic and Therapeutic

Characteristics ···················· 132

Section Three   Typical Cases ···················· 166

Chapter Two   Jiao Shude's Experience ············ 172

Section One   Understanding of Etiology and

Pathogenesis ······················ 172

Section Two   Diagnostic and Therapeutic

Characteristics ···················· 176

Section Three   Typical Cases ···················· 196

Chapter Three   Deng Tietao's Experience ········ 208

Section One   Understanding of Etiology and

Pathogenesis ······················ 208

Section Two   Diagnostic and Therapeutic

Characteristics ···················· 210

Section Three   Typical Cases ···················· 220

Index ·· 228

目　录

上篇　总　论

一、概述 ……………………………………………… 3

二、诊断要点 ………………………………………… 5

三、中医学对本病的认识 ………………………… 13

中篇　特色疗法

一、高血压病的治疗 ……………………………… 21

　（一）内治疗法 ………………………………… 21

　（二）外治疗法 ………………………………… 41

　（三）针灸疗法 ………………………………… 45

　（四）推拿疗法 ………………………………… 51

　（五）体育疗法 ………………………………… 53

　（六）情志疗法 ………………………………… 57

　（七）饮食疗法 ………………………………… 59

二、老年高血压病的治疗 ………………………… 75

　（一）六要 ……………………………………… 83

　（二）十三不要 ………………………………… 85

三、高血压病主症的治疗 ………………………… 91

　（一）头痛 ……………………………………… 91

　（二）眩晕 ……………………………………… 93

高血压病的中医特色疗法

（三）心悸 ································· 97

（四）肢麻 ································· 99

四、高血压病并发症的治疗 ·············· 103

（一）高血压脑病 ················· 103

（二）高血压危象 ················· 111

五、高血压病的摄生调护 ·············· 117

（一）减轻体重 ················· 117

（二）限制盐的摄入 ············· 119

（三）戒烟、少饮酒 ············· 119

（四）起居有常 ················· 121

下篇　名老中医治验

一、周仲瑛治验 ························· 123

（一）病机新识 ················· 123

（二）诊疗特色 ················· 133

（三）验案举隅 ················· 167

二、焦树德治验 ························· 173

（一）病机新识 ················· 173

（二）诊疗特色 ················· 177

（三）验案举隅 ················· 197

三、邓铁涛治验 ························· 209

（一）病机新识 ················· 209

（二）诊疗特色 ················· 211

（三）验案举隅 ················· 221

索引 ································· 229

Typical TCM Therapy for Primary Hypertension

高血压病的中医特色疗法

Part One   General Introduction

Chapter One   A Brief Account

Primary hypertension is a kind of independent disease with still unknown cause. It is the most common disease of the cardiovascular system, mainly manifested as elevated arterial pressure of systemic circulation, having a high morbidity. From 1979 to 1980, a survey was conducted in 29 provinces, autonomous regions and cities on 4,012,128 people aged 15 and older, which showed that the morbidity of identified hypertension was 4.85% and that of borderline hypertension was 2.88%, the total morbidity being 7.70%. In 1991, another survey was carried out on 950,356 people aged 15 and older, showing that the total morbidity of hypertension was 11.88%, 6.62% and 5.26% for identified hypertension and borderline hypertension respectively. And it is reported that at present, there are about 100 million people with hypertension in China. Clinically the disease may induce some complications of the heart, brain and kidney and is one of the leading causes of cerebral apoplexy, coronary heart

上篇 总 论

一、概述

　　高血压病是以体循环动脉压升高为主要临床表现而病因尚未明确的独立性疾病,又称原发性高血压。高血压病是最常见的心血管疾病,患病率较高。据 1979～1980 年全国 29 个省、市、自治区对 15 岁以上共 4 012 128 人的调查,确诊高血压患病率为 4.85%,临界高血压患病率为 2.88%,总患病率为 7.70%。1991 年又对 15 岁以上 950 356 人进行了调查,结果显示高血压患病率为 11.88%,其中确诊的占 6.62%,临界高血压占 5.26%。据悉,我国目前高血压病患者约 1 亿。本病还可引起严重的心、脑、肾并发症,是脑卒中、冠心病、肾功能不全的主要危险因素之一。根据起病的缓急及病程的长短可分为缓进型和急进型两型,急进

高血压病的中医特色疗法

disease and renal insufficiency. According to the onset and the courses of the disease, it is classified into lingering hypertension and acute hypertension, and the latter is also called malignant hypertension, usually having unfavourable prognosis.

Chapter Two   Diagnostic Essentials

Hypertension is a disease with gradual onset and with no symptoms at the early stage. The cases, usually at the age of 40 to 50, are accidentally found suffering from high blood pressure in physical examination. Some cases may have such symptoms as dizziness, headache, dim eyesight, tinnitus, insomnia, lassitude, etc. Upon physical examination, the aortic second sound is accentuated and in elderly cases metallic sound may be heard. Besides, there may be the fourth heart sound and aortic early systolic ejection sound. In the cases of prolonged hypertension, there appears left ventricular hypertrophy.

According to the standard of World Health Organization/World Hypertension League, with no anti-hypertensive drugs taken, hypertension is diagnosed with systolic pressure (SP)$\geqslant$18.7 kPa and/or diastolic pressure (DP)$\geqslant$12.0 kPa. The stages: Stage 1, SP$\geqslant$18.7 – 21.2 kPa and/or DP$\geqslant$12.0 –13.2 kPa; Borderline, SP$\geqslant$

型又称恶性高血压,预后多不良。

二、诊断要点

高血压病起病缓慢,早期多无症状,一般在 40～50 岁偶于体格检查时发现血压升高,有的患者可有头晕、头痛、眼花、耳鸣、失眠、乏力等症状。体检时,可听到主动脉瓣第二音亢进,年龄大者可呈金属音,可有第四心音和主动脉收缩早期喷射音。高血压持续时间长时,有左心室肥厚征象。

依据 1999 年世界卫生组织(WHO)/国际高血压联盟高血压诊断标准,高血压是指在未服用抗高血压药物的情况下,收缩压≥18.7 kPa和(或)舒张压≥12.0 kPa。其分级:若收缩压≥18.7～21.2 kPa 和(或)

18.7 –19.9 kPa and/or DP≥12.0 –12.5 kPa; Stage 2, SP≥21.3 –23.9 kPa and/or DP≥13.3 –14.5 kPa; Stage 3, SP≥24.0 kPa and/or DP≥14.7 kPa. In the case of SP>18.7 kPa, DP<12.0 kPa, it is diagnosed as simple systolic hypertension; in the case of SP≥18.7 –19.9 kPa, DP<12.0 kPa, subgroup of simple systolic hypertension. As for accelerated (malignant) hypertension, it progresses rapidly, with a persistent SP > 17.3 kPa, fundus bleeding and oozing, or papilledema, and there may appear severe damage of the heart, brain and kidney, even death.

Laboratory tests:

(1) Routine urine examination: Usually normal at the early stage, but albumen, erythrocyte and occasionally cast are found in the urine when the kidney function is impaired.

(2) Blood creatinine concentration: Increased when the kidney function is impaired.

(3) Chest radiography indicates that there is some change in the appearance and size of the heart, and in the

舒张压≥12.0～13.2 kPa 的为 1 级高血压,收缩压≥18.7～19.9 kPa 和(或)舒张压≥12.0～12.5 kPa 为临界高血压,收缩压≥21.3～23.9 kPa 和(或)舒张压≥13.3～14.5 kPa 的为 2 级高血压,收缩压≥24.0 kPa 和(或)舒张压≥14.7 kPa 的为 3 级高血压。若收缩压＞18.7 kPa,舒张压＜12.0 kPa 的为单纯收缩性高血压,收缩压≥18.7～19.9 kPa,舒张压＜12.0 kPa 的为单纯收缩性高血压的亚组。急进性(恶性)高血压病情多急骤发展,舒张压常持续在17.3 kPa以上,可有眼底出血、渗出或视神经乳头水肿,短时间内可出现心、脑、肾的严重损害,甚至危及生命。

主要实验室检查项目有:

(1)尿常规:早期病人尿常规多正常,肾功能受损时,尿中可出现蛋白、红细胞,偶见管型。

(2)血肌酐浓度:肾功能受损时可增高。

(3)胸部 X 线摄片可显示心脏外形和大小、主动脉宽度和密度(钙

width and density (calcification) of the aorta.

(4) Echocardiogram is a reliable means for the evaluation of left ventricular hypertrophy.

(5) Electrocardiographic examination discloses the involvement of the heart (hypertrophy, ischemia and infarction) and arrhythmia.

Attention should be drawn to the differentiation of primary hypertension and secondary hypertension. Usually secondary hypertension is induced by the following diseases:

(1) Diseases of renal parenchyma, for instance, glomerular nephritis, chronic nephropyelitis and polycystic kidney, with the change of urine occurring before the presence of elevated blood pressure and with rather serious impairment of kidney function. For the diagnosis, pyelography, midstream urine culture and B-type ultrasonic examination of the kidney are usually recommended.

(2) Pathologic change of the renal artery, including renal arteritis, aneurysm of renal artery and deformity of renal artery. Patients with these diseases may have hypertension at their thirties with rapid onset and deterioration. In these cases, the routine urine examination and renal function test show no abnormality, and DP is elevated obviously, but anti-hypertensive drugs do not work. Furthermore, in 50 percent of these patients, vascular

化)的变化。

(4)超声心动图为评价左心室肥厚的一个可靠的方法。

(5)心电图检查可发现由于高血压所致的心脏受累(左心室肥厚和劳损、缺血和梗死)和心律失常。

原发性高血压要与继发性高血压相鉴别。引起继发性高血压的常见疾病有：

(1)肾实质性疾病,如肾小球肾炎、慢性肾盂肾炎、多囊肾等,尿的改变出现在高血压之前,多有肾功能损害且较严重,肾盂造影、中段尿培养、肾脏B超均有助诊断。

(2)肾动脉病变,包括肾动脉炎、肾动脉瘤、肾动脉畸形等,高血压起病迅速,常急骤恶化,多于30岁以内发病。尿常规与肾功能常无明显异常,舒张压升高常特别明显,降压药效果不佳,约50%在脊肋角及上腹部两侧闻及血管杂音。核素肾图、静脉肾盂造影可显示异常,肾动脉造影可

murmurs are audible in vertebrocostal angle and bilateral epigastrium. Abnormality is found in nuclein renogram and intra-venous pyelography and confirmed diagnosis may be made by renal arterigraphy.

（3）Pheochromocytoma. Patients with this disease begin having hypertension at a younger age with intermittent elevation of blood pressure, usually SP>26.7 kPa, and sometimes with idiopathic syncope, which is manifested as headache, dizziness, pale complexion, cold extremities, severe palpitation, profuse sweating and lassitude. Urine catecholamine in 24 hours may be times of the normal level, 3-methoxy-4-hydroxy mandelic acid in urine increases and a tumor may be found by introvenous pyelography, CT scanning and B-type ultrasonic examination.

（4）Primary aldosteronism. This disease is mostly seen in female adults with manifestations as periodical weakness and paralysis of extremities, diuresis with urine of low specific gravity, also there appear hypokalemic and hypernatremic alkalosis, and increased excretion of urinary aldosterone. Retroperitoneal pneumography, adrenal venography and CT scanning are also recommended in the orientation of the tumor.

（5）Cushing's syndrome. This mostly occurs in females with the manifestations as progressive concentric obesity,

确诊。

　　(3) 嗜铬细胞瘤,发病年龄较轻,阵发性血压升高,常极高,收缩压常高于 26.7 kPa,有时出现不明原因的晕厥。症状发作时头痛且晕,面色苍白,肢凉,剧烈心悸,汗出乏力。24 小时尿儿茶酚胺可为正常数倍,尿中3-甲氧基-4-羟基苦杏仁酸升高,静脉肾盂造影、CT 扫描、B 超发现瘤体可以确诊。

　　(4) 原发性醛固酮增多症,多发于成年女性,除血压升高外,有周期性四肢无力、麻痹等神经肌肉症状及多尿、尿比重降低等,血电解质显示低血钾、高血钠性碱中毒,尿醛固酮排泄量增多。腹膜后充气造影、肾上腺静脉造影、CT 扫描对肿瘤定位有重要帮助。

　　(5) 库欣综合征,多发于女性,患者呈进行性向心性肥胖,面色红润,

flushed face, purple-striae skin, increased excretion of free cortisol and 17 - hydroxy-cortisol in 24 hours and increase of blood cortisol. ACTH excitation test, DXM suppression test, radiography of sellar turcica region, intravenous pyelography and retroperitoneal pneumography are helpful in making the diagnosis of the disease.

Chapter Three   Understanding of Primary Hypertension in TCM

In TCM, primary hypertension is recognized as "dizziness", "headache", "liver-yang", "liver-wind", etc., and especially as the former two. Through the ages, practitioners have had profound and detailed analyses of manifestations, etiology, pathogenesis, diagnosis and treatment of the disease.

Main causes of primary hypertension:

(1) Emotional upsets: Excessive anger, long-term anxiety, terror, strain or emotional liability, impairs the liver's ability to promote the free flow of qi and turns stagnant liver-qi into fire, leading to flaming up of liver-fire and hyperactivity of liver-yang, thus headache occurs.

(2) Improper diet: Immoderate eating, intake of heavy greasy food or excessive drinking impairs the spleen and stomach, causing dampness to produce. Prolonged reten-

皮肤出现紫纹,24 小时游离皮质醇与尿 17 - 羟皮质醇排泄量增多,血皮质醇增高,ACTH 兴奋试验、地塞米松抑制试验、蝶鞍摄片、静脉肾盂造影与腹膜后充气造影均有助于诊断。

三、中医学对本病的认识

在中医学中,有关高血压病的认识多散见在"眩晕"、"头痛"、"肝阳"、"肝风"等疾病名中,尤以眩晕、头痛为主来认识。对眩晕和头痛,历代医家都有深刻的认识,对症状表现、病因病机和诊治等均作了详细的分析。

本病的主要病因有:

(1)情志失调:过度恼怒、长期忧思及恐惧紧张和情绪波动,使肝气郁滞,肝气郁久而化为肝火,肝火上炎,肝阳上亢发为本病。

(2)饮食不节:饥饱失常,或过食肥甘厚味,或饮酒无度,皆可损伤脾胃,以致湿浊内生,湿浊日久化热,

tion of dampness turns to heat and then produces phlegm, which blocks the meridians. Subsequently lucid yang fails to ascend and turbid yin fails to descend, leading to dysfunction of qi and failure of lucid yang to nourish orifices, thus headache occurs.

(3) Prolonged illness and overstrain: Prolonged illness or overstrain impairs healthy qi of the body, causing deficiency or imbalance of yin and yang and hypofunction of viscera. In this case, accumulation of metabolites in the body brings dizziness and headache, thus giving rise to hypertension. In cases of excessive mental activity causing consumption of blood, weakness due to old age, excessive sexual activity leading to consumption of kidney essence, or postpartum deficiency of qi and blood, essence and blood are deficient. Since the liver and kidney have the same origin, if kidney-essence fails to nourish liver-yin, deficient liver-yin fails to suppress yang, resulting in hyperactivity of liver-yang and endogenous deficient wind. As a result, headache occurs.

Pathogenesis:

(1) Hyperactivity of liver-yang: In the case of yang excess and yin deficiency, yin and yang lose their balance, with deficient yin in the lower and hyperactive yang in the upper; prolonged stress or anxiety, depression, anger impairs the liver function, causing stagnation

热灼津液成痰,痰浊阻滞经络,使清阳不升,浊阴不降,气机失常,清窍失养或痰热上蒙清窍而发为本病。

(3)久病过劳:久病和过劳常可伤及人体正气,使阴阳偏衰、失调,脏腑、气血功能低下,体内代谢产物积聚而出现头晕、头痛,产生高血压病。如劳神过度,暗耗心血,或年老体虚,或房室不节,肾精亏损,或妇人产后气血损伤,均可导致精血亏虚。而肝肾同源,肾精不养肝阴,则肝阴不足,阴不敛阳,肝阳偏亢,虚风内动,而发为本病。

本病的主要病机有:

(1)肝阳上亢:素体阳盛阴衰之人,阴阳平衡失其常度,阴亏于下,阳亢于上;长期精神紧张或忧思郁怒,使肝失条达,肝气郁结,气郁化火伤阴,肝阴耗伤,风阳易动,上扰头目;

of liver-qi which turns to fire and consumes liver-yin, and then wind-yang disturbs the head; in the case of deficient kidney-yin failing to nourish the liver, kidney (water) is prevented from nourishing liver (wood), leading to hyperactivity of liver-yang. In the above-said cases, dizziness, headache and hypertension may appear.

(2) Deficiency of liver-yin and kidney-yin: Liver-yin and kidney-yin influence each other. Deficiency of kidney-yin leads to deficiency of liver-yin, and vice versa. When deficient liver-yin and kidney-yin fail to suppress yang, hyperactive yang rushes upward and hypertension is produced.

(3) Deficiency of yin and yang: Prolonged diseases usually impair yin and yang. In most of the hypertension cases, there appears yin impairing yang and ultimately deficiency of both yin and yang, which is especially seen in those at the later stage and accompanied with renal failure due to kidney damage.

(4) Internal stagnation of phlegm: Improper diet or over-intake of greasy food impairs the spleen and stomach; anxiety or over fatigue impairs the spleen leading to failure of the spleen in transportation, then dampness stagnation appears and phlegm is produced; stagnant liver-qi results in retention of dampness and phlegm is produced. Consequently the phlegm blocks the meridians, or sometimes with the presence of endogenous wind, which is manifested as headache or

或肾阴素亏不能养肝,水不涵木,而致肝阳上亢等,均可出现眩晕、头痛,产生高血压。

(2)肝肾阴虚:肝肾阴虚常互为因果,肾阴不足可导致肝阴不足,相反肝阴不足亦可致肾阴不足。肝肾阴虚,不能涵敛阳气,阳气亢逆上冲,可形成高血压。

(3)阴阳两虚:多因病久不愈,阴阳俱损而致。在高血压病患者中多见阴损及阳,最终阴阳两虚。这种病机多见高血压病后期患者,尤其是伴有肾脏损害而引起肾功能衰竭者,常表现出阴阳两虚的病机变化。

(4)痰浊内阻:饮食不节,过食肥甘厚味,损伤脾胃,或忧思、劳倦伤脾,以致脾虚健运失职,水湿内停,积聚成痰;或肝气郁结,气郁湿滞而生痰。痰阻经络,或兼内生之风火作祟,则表现头痛,眩晕欲仆。临床上多见于高血压脑部病变严重患者。

ر

dizziness and mostly seen in severe cases with cerebral lesion due to hypertension.

(5) Imbalance of both thoroughfare and conception vessels: In climacteric, deficient kidney-yin causes imbalance of both thoroughfare and conception vessels, especially in the cases of deficiency of liver-yin and kidney-yin and this imbalance leads to deficiency and disorder of qi and blood, resulting in hypertension.

(6) Blockage of blood stasis in the collaterals: As it is recorded in the Chinese medical classics, "New cases usually appear in channels while prolonged ones involve collaterals", or "New cases usually appear in qifen while prolonged ones involve xuefen". Blood stasis in the collaterals may be seen in the later stage of hypertension with its clinical manifestations as unsmooth pulse, cyanosis, ecchymosis, and pain, etc.

To sum up, hypertension, which is considered as an excess-deficiency imbalance in TCM, is mostly related to the liver, kidney and heart, with imbalance between yin and yang as its primary cause and wind, fire, phlegm, blood stasis as its secondary causes. Among the cases of hypertension, the new cases, the young and the middle-aged are attributed to excess type while the prolonged and the aged ones are characterized by primary deficiency and secondary excess.

（5）冲任失调：随着年龄的增大，进入更年期，肾中精气亏虚，便可引起冲任失调。而素有肝肾之阴不足的人则更易在更年期发生冲任失调。冲任失调，则气血虚损、逆乱，形成高血压病。

（6）瘀血阻络："初病在经，久病入络"、"初病在气，久病入血"，后期高血压病常可见瘀血阻络的病机，临床表现为脉涩、紫绀、瘀斑、疼痛等。

综上所述，高血压病主要病位在肝、肾、心，病之本为阴阳失调，病之标为风、火、痰、瘀，是虚实相兼的疾病。中青年人和新病者多为实证，老年人和久病者多为本虚标实。

Part Two   Distinctive Treatment

Chapter One   Treatment of Primary Hypertension

Section One   Internal Treatment

1. Syndrome differentiation and Treatment

Primary hypertension is a kind of disease with wind, fire, phlegm and blood stasis as its secondary causes and with deficiency of the liver and kidney as its primary cause. Clinically, the disease is characterized by deficiency syndrome predominant over excess syndrome, yin deficiency over yang deficiency. But in woman cases, it mostly results from dysfunction of thoroughfare and conception vessels. Therefore treatment should be adopted according to individual cases and as for the complicated ones, different causes should be taken into account in dealing with the disease.

(1) Hyperactivity of liver-yang

Chief manifestations: Distending pain of the head, dizziness, flushed face, irritability, tinnitus, deafness,

中篇 特色疗法

一、高血压病的治疗

（一）内治疗法

1. 辨证治疗

本病以风、火、痰、瘀为标，肝肾亏虚为本。从临床实践看来，本病虚证多于实证，阴虚多于阳虚。妇女高血压病，则多与冲任失调有关。故在治疗上各有所侧重，而对于错杂之病，则应多方兼顾。

（1）肝阳上亢

【证候】 头目胀痛，眩晕，面红目赤，烦躁易怒，耳鸣耳聋，口苦舌

bitter taste in the mouth, dryness of the tongue, dark urine, constipation; red tongue with thick, yellow, or greasy yellow coating; wiry, rapid and forceful pulse.

Therapeutic principle: Calm the liver and suppress yang, clear away heat and subdue fire.

Prescription: Modified Longdan Xiegan Tang (decoction), composed of Longdancao 6 – 10 g, Juhua 10 g, Huangqin 10 g, Zhizi 10 g, Zexie 10 – 15 g, Caojueming 15 – 30 g, Shengdihuang 12 – 20 g, Zhidahuang 3 – 10 g, Mudanpi 10 g and Gouteng 10 – 30 g (decocted later).

Modification: For the case with severe headache and dizziness, add Zhenzhumu (decocted first) 30 g and Shengshijueming (decocted first) 30 g; for numbness of extremities, add Guangdilong 10 – 12 g; for rigidity of nape, add Gegen 15 – 20 g.

(2) Deficiency of yin and hyperactivity of yang

Chief manifestations: Headache, dizziness, tinnitus, dim eyesight, heaviness of the head, palpitation, insomnia, restlessness, dreaminess, lassitude of the waist and knees, dry mouth and throat; red tongue with little or thin yellow coating; wiry, small and rapid pulse.

Therapeutic principle: Nourish yin and calm the liver.

Prescription: Modified Tianma Gouteng Yin (decoction) and Qiju Dihuang Wan (pill), composed of Tianma 10 g, Gouteng 10 – 13 g (decocted later), Shengshijue-

干,尿赤便结。舌质红,苔黄厚或黄
腻,脉弦数有力。

【治法】 平肝潜阳,清热降火。

【方药】 龙胆泻肝汤加减。龙胆
草 6～10 g,菊花10 g,黄芩10 g,栀子
10 g,泽泻 10～15 g,草决明15～30 g,生
地黄 12～20 g,制大黄 3～10 g,牡丹皮
10 g,钩藤(后下)10～30 g。

【加减】 头痛眩晕甚者加珍珠
母(先煎)30 g,生石决明(先煎)30 g;
肢麻加广地龙 10～12 g;头项强痛加
葛根 15～20 g。

(2) 阴虚阳亢

【证候】 头痛眩晕,耳鸣眼花,
头重脚轻,心悸失眠,心烦多梦,腰膝
酸软,咽干口燥。舌红苔少或薄黄,
脉弦细数。

【治法】 滋阴平肝。

【方药】 天麻钩藤饮合杞菊地
黄丸加减:天麻10 g,钩藤（后下）
10～30 g,生石决明(先煎)20～30 g,

ming 20 – 30 g (decocted first), Chuanniuxi 10 – 15 g, Sangjisheng 15 –30 g, Fushen 15 –30 g, Shengdihuang 15 – 30 g, Baijuhua 12 g, Gegen 15 –20 g and Shanzhuyu 12 g.

Modification: For severe lumbago, add Duzhong 10 – 12 g; for dry mouth, add Shihu 10 –12 g; for dry stool, add Huomaren 10 g; for numbness of extremities, add Xixiancao 15 –30 g and Luoshiteng 15 –30 g.

(3) Internal abundance of phlegm

Chief manifestations: Dizziness, headache, heaviness of the head, fullness in the chest and epigastrium, anorexia and nausea, palpitation, edema, weakness of extremeties; greasy white or greasy yellow tongue coating, small and smooth pulse.

Therapeutic principle: Resolve phlegm to suppress wind.

Prescription: Modified Banxia Baizhu Tianma Tang (decoction), composed of Fabanxia 10 g, Baizhu 12 g, Tianma 6 g, Fuling 15 g, Chenpi 10 g, Gouteng 15 g (decocted later), Shichangpu 10 g, Zhike 10 g and Gancao 6 g.

Modification: For the complicated cases with dizziness, chest distress and epigastric flatulence, profuse sputum, and numbness of extremeties, add Beimu 10 g, Tianzhuhuang 6 g and Huangqin 10 g; for scanty urine, add Cheqiancao 15 –20 g; for dominant dampness-heat of

川牛膝 10～15 g,桑寄生 15～30 g,茯神 15～30 g,生地黄 15～30 g,白菊花 12 g,葛根 15～20 g,山茱萸 12 g。

【加减】 腰痛甚加杜仲 10～12 g;口干加石斛 10～12 g;大便干结加火麻仁 10 g;肢麻可加豨莶草 15～30 g,络石藤 15～30 g。

(3) 痰湿内盛

【证候】 头晕头痛,头重如裹,胸闷脘胀,食少欲吐,心悸浮肿,四肢无力。舌苔白腻或黄腻,脉细滑。

【治法】 化痰熄风。

【方药】 半夏白术天麻汤加味。法半夏 10 g,白术 12 g,天麻 6 g,茯苓 15 g,陈皮 10 g,钩藤(后下)15 g,石菖蒲 10 g,枳壳 10 g,甘草 6 g。

【加减】 头晕、胸闷、痰多、肢体麻木者加贝母 10 g,天竺黄 6 g,黄芩 10 g;尿少加车前草 15～20 g;肝胆湿热明显加茵陈 10～12 g,黄芩 10～15 g。

the liver and gallbladder, add Yinchen 10 - 12 g and Huangqin 10 -15 g.

(4) Deficiency of Yin and Yang

Chief manifestations: Dizziness, lassitude of the waist and legs, tinnitus, deafness, palpitation, insomnia, shortness of breath when moving, cold and numb limbs, frequent urination at night or yin-cold impotence; pale tongue with clean coating, small and weak, or slow intermittent pulse.

Therapeutic principle: Replenish yin and invigorate yang.

Prescription: Modified Erxian Tang (decoction) and Jinkui Shenqi Wan (pill), composed of Xianmao 12 g, Xianlingpi 12 g, Bajitian 12 g, Gouqizi 12 g, Shanzhuyu 12 g, Gandihuang 24 g, Shudihuang 15 - 30 g, Mudanpi 10 g, Zhimu 10 g, Danggui 10 g, Wuweizi 6 g and Shengmuli (decocted first) 30 g.

Modification: For deficiency of kidney-yang, add Paofuzi 3 -10 g and Rougui (decocted later) 3 g; for deficiency of the spleen, add Fuling 15 -20 g and Baizhu 9 - 15 g; for deficiency of qi, add Huangqi 30 -45 g; for frequent urination, add Yizhiren and Buguzhi 10 g respectively.

(5) Dysfunction of thoroughfare and conception vessels

（4）阴阳两虚

【证候】　头目眩晕,腰酸腿软,耳聋耳鸣,心悸健忘,动则气促,肢凉麻木,夜尿频数,或见阴冷阳痿。舌淡苔净,脉细弱或结代。

【治法】　益阴助阳。

【方药】　二仙汤合金匮肾气丸加减。仙茅12 g,仙灵脾12 g,巴戟天12 g,枸杞子12 g,山茱萸12 g,干地黄24 g,熟地黄 15～30 g,牡丹皮10 g,知母10 g,当归10 g,五味子6 g,生牡蛎(先煎)30 g。

【加减】　肾阳虚者加炮附子3～10 g,肉桂（后下）3 g;脾虚加茯苓15～20 g,白术 9～15 g;气虚明显加黄芪 30～45 g;尿频数加益智仁、补骨脂各10 g。

（5）冲任失调

Chief manifestations: Headache, dizziness, restlessness, insomnia, tinnitus, irritability, feverish sensation in the palms and soles, amnesia, shortness of breath, menstrual disorder; red tongue with thin coating, wiry and small pulse.

Therapeutic principle: Regulate thoroughfare and conception vessels.

Prescription: Modified Erxian Tang (decoction), composed of Xianmao 10 g, Xianlingpi 12 g, Chishaoyao 12 g, Baishaoyao 12 g, Bajitian 12 g, Danggui 15 g, Zhimu 10 g, and Huangbai 10 g.

Modification: For severe cases of dizziness, add Gouteng 12 g (decocted later); for restlessness and insomnia, add Suanzaoren 15 g, Yejiaoteng 12 g and Baiziren 10 g; for irritability, add Chaihu 10 g and Zisugeng 10 g; for dizziness and distention of the head, add Xiakucao 12 g.

2. Chinese patent medicine

(1) Niuhuang Qingxin Wan (bolus) (*Experience in Treating Eruptive Diseases*)

Composition: Niuhuang, Zhusha, Huanglian, Huangqin, Zhizi and Yujin.

Indications: Applicable to cases of hyperactivity of liver-yang or dizziness and headache due to accumulation of phlegm-fire.

【证候】 头晕头痛,心烦失眠,耳鸣易怒,手足心热,记忆力减退,心慌气短,月经失调。舌红苔薄,脉弦细。

【治法】 调补冲任。

【方药】 二仙汤加味。仙茅10 g,仙灵脾12 g,赤芍药、白芍药各12 g,巴戟天12 g,当归15 g,知母10 g,黄柏10 g。

【加减】 头晕甚者加钩藤(后下)12 g;心烦不寐者加酸枣仁15 g,夜交藤12 g,柏子仁10 g;烦躁易怒加柴胡10 g,紫苏梗10 g;头晕头胀加夏枯草12 g。

2. 中成药

(1) 牛黄清心丸(《痘疹世医心法》)

【组成】 牛黄、朱砂、黄连、黄芩、栀子、郁金。

【适应证】 肝阳上亢及痰火壅盛致眩晕头痛。

Administration: One bolus each time, twice daily, taken with boiled water.

(2) Niuhuang Jiangya Wan (bolus) (*Hubei Province Criteria for Drugs*, 1985 Ed.)

Composition: Lingyangjiao, Zhenzhumu, Niuhuang, Bingpian, Huangqi and Yujin.

Indications: Applicable to hyperactivity of liver-yang.

Administration: One bolus each time, twice daily.

(3) Naoliqing (pill) (*Beijing Criteria for Drugs*, 1983 Ed.)

Composition: Cishi, Daizheshi, Huainiuqi, Qing-banxia, Jiuqu, Zhenzhumu, Bohe wine, Bingpian and Danfen.

Indications: Applicable to hyperactivity of liver-yang.

Administration: 10 pills each time, twice daily; con-traindicated for pregnant woman and cases of deficiency-cold.

(4) Quantianma Jiaonang (capsule) (*Guizhou Yikang Pharmaceutical* CO., LTD.)

Composition: Tianma only.

Indications: Applicable to hyperactivity of liver-yang with stirring-up of liver-wind.

Administration: 4 capsules each time, 3 times daily.

【服法】　每日 2 次,每次 1 丸,白开水送服。

(2)牛黄降压丸(《河北省药品标准》1985 年版)

【组成】　羚羊角、珍珠母、牛黄、冰片、黄芪、郁金。

【适应证】　高血压肝阳上亢型。

【服法】　每日服 2 次,每次 1 丸。

(3)脑立清(《北京市药品标准》1983 年版)

【组成】　磁石、代赭石、怀牛膝、清半夏、酒曲、珍珠母、薄荷酒、冰片、胆粉。

【适应证】　高血压肝阳上亢型。

【服法】　每次 10 粒,每日 2 次。孕妇忌服。体弱虚寒者不宜使用。

(4)全天麻胶囊(贵州益康制药有限公司)

【组成】　天麻。

【适应证】　高血压肝阳上亢,肝风上扰型。

【服法】　每次服 4 粒,每日 3 次。

(5) Shanlücha Jiangya   Pian (tablet) (*Guangxi Guilin Pharmaceutical Factory*)

Composition: Shanlücha and others.

Indications: Applicable to hyperactivity of liver-yang with stirring up of liver-wind.

Administration: 3 tablets each time, 3 times daily.

(6) Qiju Dihuang Ye (oral liquid) (*Comprehensive Medical Collections*)

Composition: Gouqizi, Juhua, Shudihuang, Shanyao, Shanzhuyu, Zexie, Mudanpi and Fuling.

Indications: Applicable to deficiency of liver-yin and kidney-yin.

Administration: One vial each time, 3 times daily.

(7) Tianma Shouwu Pian (tablet) (*Hunan Province Criteria for Drugs*, 1989 Ed.)

Composition: Tianma, Heshouwu, Chuanwu, Mohanlian and Cijili, etc..

Indications: Applicable to deficiency of liver-yin and kidney-yin.

Administration: 6 tablets a time, 3 times daily.

3. Simple prescription and experiential prescription

(1) Jiangya Jiaonang (capsule)

Composition: Nüzhenzi, Hanliancao, Cishi, Huai-

（5）山绿茶降压片（广西桂林制药厂）

【组成】　山绿茶等。

【适应证】　高血压肝阳上亢，肝风上扰型。

【服法】　每次服 3 片，每日 3 次。

（6）杞菊地黄液（《医级》）

【组成】　枸杞子、菊花、熟地黄、山药、山茱萸、泽泻、牡丹皮、茯苓。

【适应证】　高血压肝肾阴虚型。

【服法】　每次服 1 支，每日 3 次。

（7）天麻首乌片（《湖南省药品标准》1989 年版）

【组成】　天麻、何首乌、川乌、墨旱莲、刺蒺藜等。

【适应证】　高血压肝肾阴虚型。

【服法】　每次服 6 片，每日 3 次。

3. 单方验方

（1）降压胶囊

【组成】　女贞子、旱莲草、磁石、

niuxi, Dahuang, Xiakucao and Fenfangji.

Procedure: Decoct with water all the herbs except Fenfangji and concentrate the decoction into extract, then dry the extract with powdered Fangji, fill capsules with the mixture, one capsule containing 0.25 g.

Administration: 2 – 4 capsules a day, 3 times daily, 30 days as a course of treatment.

Actions: Nourish the liver and kidney and suppress fire.

(2) Xiakucao Tangjiang (syrup)

Composition: Xiakucao 120 g, Caojueming 100 g and white sugar 120 g.

Procedure: Add 2,000 ml of water to Xiakucao and Caojueming in an earthen pot, decoct the herbs on a slow fire to 1,500 ml; filter the decoction with gauze, decoct the dregs with water, then mix the decoction with white sugar and stir, the syrup is thus produced.

Administration: 300 ml each time, 3 times daily, 30 days as a course of treatment.

Actions: Clear away liver-fire and gallbladder-fire, promote diuresis, lower blood pressure, lower blood-lipid, also nourish the liver and invigorate the spleen, raise lucid yang and lower turbid substance, and used as a preventive against apoplexy.

(3) Pingjiang Tang (decoction)

Composition: Zexie 60 g, Yimucao 30 g, Huainiuxi

怀牛膝、大黄、夏枯草、粉防己。

【制法】　前 6 味药水煎后浓缩成膏,加粉防己粉烘干,装胶囊,每粒 0.25 g。

【服法】　每次 2～4 粒,每日 3 次,30 日为 1 个疗程。

【功用】　滋补肝肾,潜镇降火。

(2) 夏枯草糖浆

【组成】　夏枯草120 g,草决明 100 g,白糖120 g。

【制法】　先将夏枯草、草决明放入沙锅内,加清水2 000 ml,文火煎至 1 500 ml时,用纱布过滤,药渣加水再煎,最后将汁混合在一起加入白糖,搅拌溶化后即成。此为 3 日量。

【服法】　每次 300 ml,每日 3 次,30 日为 1 个疗程。

【功用】　清肝利胆,利尿降压,降血脂。且有保肝健脾,升清降浊,预防中风的作用。

(3) 平降汤

【组成】　泽泻60 g,益母草30 g,

15 g, Gouteng 15 g (decocted later), Xiakucao 15 g, Sangjisheng 15 g, Shengshijueming 30 g (decocted first), and Tianma 10 g.

Procedure: Decoct Shengshijueming with water first for 30 minutes or more, add the other herbs except Gouteng, simmer for 40 minutes, then add Gouteng, simmer for another 5 - 10 minutes, take the dregs out when the decoction is still hot and add the melted drug; one dose a day, each dose being decocted two times to get 500 ml of decoction.

Administration: 250ml each time after meals in the morning and evening, 20 days as a course of treatment.

Actions: Nourish the liver and kidney, calm the liver and suppress yang, clear away heat and promote diuresis.

(4) Fufang Huaihua Jiangya Tang (decoction)

Composition: Huaihua 25 g, Sangjisheng 25 g, Chuanxiong 15 g and Dilong 15 g.

Administration: Decoct the herbs with water, one dose a day.

Actions: Disperse stagnated liver-qi to promote blood circulation, nourish yin and suppress yang; applicable to hypertension with stagnation of liver-qi and blood stasis and hyperactivity of yang due to deficiency of liver-yin and kidney-yin.

(5) Jiangya Fang (decoction)

怀牛膝15 g,钩藤(后下)15 g,夏枯草15 g,桑寄生15 g,生石决明(先煎)30 g,天麻10 g。

【制法】 水煎服,煎时将先煎的药物先煎30分钟以上,再入群药,用文火煎40分钟左右,再加后入之品,煎5~10分钟即可,趁热弃去药渣,将烊化之药放入。每日1剂,每剂煎2次,共取汁500 ml。

【服法】 每次250 ml,早晚饭后服,20剂为1个疗程。

【功用】 滋补肝肾,平肝潜阳,清热利湿。

(4)复方槐花降压汤

【组成】 槐花25 g,桑寄生25 g,川芎15 g,地龙15 g。

【用法】 水煎服,每日1剂。

【功用】 疏肝活血,养阴潜阳。适用于肝郁血瘀,肝肾阴虚阳亢之高血压病患者。

(5)降压方

Composition: Shengshijueming 30 g, Luobumaye 30 g, Xixiancao 30 g, Baishaoyao 10 g, Yimucao 10 g, Fenfangji 10 g, Sangjisheng 15 g and Danshen 15 g.

Administration: Decoct the herbs with water, one dose a day.

Actions: Calm the liver and suppress yang, promote blood circulation and lower blood pressure; applicable to hypertension of different types.

(6) Fufang Huangguateng Pian (tablet)

Composition: Huangguateng and others.

Procedure: Prepare the herbs into tablets, each tablet being 0.35 g, which is equal to 2.3 g of dried Huangguateng.

Administration: Take 4 tablets each time, 3 times daily.

Actions: Lower blood pressure and lower blood-lipid, applicable to hypertension of various types.

(7) Cebaiye, Chouwutong and Sangshugen, 30 g respectively, decoct the herbs with water.

(8) Xiaojicao 30 g, Cheqiancao 30 g and Xixiancao 15 g, decoct the herbs with water.

(9) Jicai 100 g and Xianshuqucao 30 g, decoct the herbs with water.

(10) Hanqincai (with old leaves and fibrous roots removed) 2 - 3 kg, chop the herb and decoct with water,

【组成】　生石决明、罗布麻叶、稀莶草各30 g,白芍药、益母草、粉防己各10 g,桑寄生、丹参各15 g。

【用法】　水煎服,每日 1 剂。

【功用】　平肝潜阳,活血降压。适用于各型高血压病患者。

(6)复方黄瓜藤片

【组成】　黄瓜藤等。

【制法】　压片,每片0.35 g,相当于干黄瓜藤2.3 g。

【用法】　口服 4 片 1 次,每日 3 次。

【功用】　降压降脂。适用于各型高血压病患者。

(7)侧柏叶、臭梧桐、桑树根各30 g,煎服。

(8)小蓟草、车前草各30 g,稀莶草15 g,煎服。

(9)荠菜100 g,鲜鼠曲草30 g,水煎服。

(10)旱芹菜(去老叶及须)2～3 kg,切碎加水煎,入罐密封,变酸后

pour the decoction into an earthen pot; seal the pot and add in 60 –120 g of sugar when it turns sour; one bowl of the decoction every day.

(11) Luobumaye 6 –9 g, Gouteng 3 –6 g and Dazao 4 pieces, decoct the herbs with water, 2 – 3 times daily; applicable to hypertension with headache and insomnia.

(12) Lingzhi, decoct it with water, 6 –9 g a day; effective for lowering blood pressure.

(13) Juhua 9 g, decoct it with water and take the decoction, one dose daily; applicable to hypertension and also effeitive for clearing away heat to brighten vision.

(14) Yama 10 –20 g, decoct it with water, take the decoction 2 times a day; applicable to hypertension with hypercholesterolemia.

Section Two   External Therapy

1. Application method

(1) Wuzhuyu 500 g (prepared with bile), Longdan-cao 6 g (extracted with alcohol), Liuhuang 50 g, Baifan (prepared with vinegar) 100 g, Zhusha 50 g and cyclopenthi-aside 175 g. Mix the above ingredients according to their respective quantity and grind them together into fine powder. For each time, put 200 mg of the prepared powder at the navel, then cover it with a piece of soft paper and fix it with adhesive tape. Change the powder once a week and continue the

加糖 60～120 g。每日 1 次,每服 1 碗。

（11）罗布麻叶 6～9 g,钩藤 3～
6 g,大枣 4 枚,加水煎服,每日 2～3
次,用于高血压病头痛,失眠。

（12）灵芝,水煎服,每日 6～9 g。
有降压作用。

（13）菊花 9 g,水煎代茶,每日
1 剂。可治高血压病,并能清热明目。

（14）亚麻 10～20 g,水煎去渣,
日服 2 次。高血压病伴有血胆固醇
增高者较宜。

（二）外治疗法

1. 敷贴法

（1）胆汁制吴茱萸500 g,龙胆草
醇提取物 6 g,硫黄 50 g,醋制白矾
100 g,朱砂50 g,环戊甲噻嗪175 mg。
将上方按量混合研成细面,备用。每
次取 200 mg,置于脐中,外用软纸敷
盖加胶布固定,每周更换 1 次,用药 3
周左右。

treatment for about three weeks.

（2）Baihuasheshecao, Wugong, Chantui, Dilong, Zhechong, Huanglian, Baijiezi, Yanhusuo, Gegen, Gansui, Xixin and Sanqi. Grind the ingredients into fine powder, then mix it with ginger juice to make a medicinal cake and put a little musk in the middle of the cake. Apply the medicinal cake on bilateral acupoints of Xinshu （BL15）, Ganshu （BL18）, Shenshu （BL23） and Guanyuan （CV4） for 8－12 hours.

（3）Blend Wuzhuyu powder with vinegar and stick it in the middle of both soles. This application has the function of lowering high blood pressure.

2. Fumigation and washing therapy

（1）Chongweizi, Gouteng and Sangshupi. Decoct 50 g of each of the above ingredients with water, then soak the feet in the decoction for 30 minutes.

（2）Gouteng 20 g and a small amount of Bingpian. Cut Gouteng into small pieces and wrap Bingpian in a piece of cloth, put them together in a basin and add in warm water, then bathe the feet in the basin for 30－35 minutes, twice a day: once before going to bed in the evening and once after getting up in the morning, ten days being a course of treatment.

3. Medicinal pillow

（1）Bohe, Yejuhua, Qingmuxiang, Danzhuye, Sheng-

（2）白花蛇舌草、蜈蚣、蝉蜕、地龙、䗪虫、黄连、白芥子、延胡索、葛根、甘遂、细辛、三七,共研细末,拌以姜汁,做成药饼。中心放少许麝香末。将上药饼贴于两侧心俞、肝俞、肾俞及关元穴,8～12 小时取下。

（3）吴茱萸研末,醋调贴于两脚心,有降压作用。

2. 熏洗法

（1）茺蔚子、钩藤、桑树皮各50 g,煎水。用所煎药水浸泡双足 30 分钟。

（2）钩藤20 g,冰片少许。取钩藤20 g剪碎,布包冰片少许,于每日晨起和晚睡前放入盆内,并加温水浴脚,每次 30～45 分钟,早晚各 1 次,10 日为 1 个疗程。

3. 药枕

（1）薄荷,野菊花,青木香,淡竹

shigao, Baishaoyao, Chuanxiong, Dongsangye, Manjingzi, Cishi and Wancansha. Pulverize equal amount of each of the above ingredients into small pieces, then put them into a cloth bag to make a medicinal pillow. Use the pillow no less than 6 hours a day; applicable to hypertension with hyperactivity of liver-yang.

(2) Juhua, Chuanxiong, Mudanpi and Baizhi. Pulverize equal amount of each of the above ingredients into small pieces and put them into a cloth bag to make a medicinal pillow.

Section Three   Acupuncture-moxibustion Therapy

1. Body acupuncture

(1) Acupoints: Fengchi (GB20), Ganshu (BL18), Shenshu (BL23), Xingjian (LR2), Xiaxi (GB43).

Manipulation: Reducing method.

Indications: Hyperactivity of liver-yang.

(2) Acupoints: Zhongwan (CV12), Neiguan (PC6), Fenglong(ST40), Jiexi (ST41).

Manipulation: Reducing method.

Indications: Phlegm stagnation.

(3) Acupoints: Pishu (BL20), Shenshu (BL23), Guanyuan (CV4), Zusanli (ST36).

Manipulation: Reinforcing method.

Indications: Liver-deficiency and kidney-deficiency.

叶,生石膏,白芍药,川芎,冬桑叶,蔓荆子,磁石,晚蚕沙。等量粉碎后装入布袋制成药枕,每昼夜使用时间不少于 6 小时。适用于高血压肝阳上亢型。

（2）菊花,川芎,牡丹皮,白芷。将上药等量粉碎后装入布袋内制成药枕。

（三）针灸疗法

1. 体针

（1）方 1：风池、肝俞、肾俞、行间、侠溪,针法用泻法,适用于肝阳上亢证。

（2）方 2：中脘、内关、丰隆、解溪,针用泻法,适用于痰湿阻逆证。

（3）方 3：脾俞、肾俞、关元、足三里,针用补法,适用于肝肾两虚证。

高血压病的中医特色疗法

2. Ear acupuncture

Acupoints: Stomach, Ear-Shenmen, Occiput, Internal Ear, Subcortex.

Method: Use 2 - 3 acupoints each time, with moderate and strong stimulation, retain the needle for 20 - 30 minutes and rotate the needle at intervals, once a day, with 5 - 7 days as a course of treatment.

3. Scalp acupuncture

Stimulation areas: Vertigo and Audition Area (bilateral).

Method: Once a day, 5 - 10 days as a course of treatment.

4. Moxibustion

Acupoints: Zusanli (ST36), Juegu (GB39).

Method: Apply moxa cone of rice-grain size over Zusanli and Juegu, once or twice a week, 1 - 3 cones for a point (bilateral) each time, with ten times as a course of treatment.

5. Acupoint injection

(1) Hegu (LI4), Taichong (LR 3), Yiming (EX-HN14) or Neiguan (PC6), Fengchi (GB20) and Sidu (SJ9). Apply 2 - 3 points each time for 3 -5 ml of 5% or 10% glucose injection, or 0.5 ml of vitamin B_{12} injection into each point, once every other day.

(2) Quchi(LI11), Zusanli(ST36), Taichong(LR 3).

2. 耳针

【选穴】 胃、神门、枕、内耳、皮质下。

【用法】 每次取 2～3 穴,中强刺激,留针 20～30 分钟,间歇捻针。每日 1 次,5～7 日为 1 个疗程。

3. 头针

【选穴】 双侧晕听区。

【用法】 每日 1 次,5～10 次为 1 个疗程。

4. 艾灸

【选穴】 足三里、绝骨。

【用法】 用米粒大小艾炷直接灸病人足三里和绝骨,每周 1～2 次,每次 1 穴(双),每穴灸 1～3 壮,10 次为 1 个疗程。

5. 穴位注射

(1) 方 1:合谷、太冲、翳明或内关、风池、四渎。每次取 2～3 穴,每穴注射 5% 或 10% 葡萄糖液 3～5 ml,或维生素 B_{12} 注射液 0.5 ml,隔日 1 次。

(2) 方 2:曲池、足三里、太冲。

Select at random a pair of these points each time for 0. 1 - 0. 2 ml of reserpine injection into each point.

(3) Zusanli(ST36), Neiguan (PC6), Hegu (LI4), Sanyinjiao(SP6). Apply one point on the upper limb and one point on the lower limb each time and use the points in turn. Inject 1 ml of 0. 25% procaine into each point, once a day, with ten to fifteen days as a course of treatment.

6. Pricking therapy for blood-letting

The main point is Touwei (ST8). For the case with dizziness and a feeling of fullness and discomfort in the forehead, add Cuanzhu (BL2); for the case with severe chest distress and chest pain, add Yintang (EX-HN3) and Shangxing (GV23); for the case with dizziness and pain in the top of the head and forehead, add Baihui(GV20), and for the severe cases, add Sishencong (EX-HN1); add Fengchi (GB 20) for the patient with dizziness accompanied by stiff neck; add temple for the patient feeling dizzy and likely to fall down. Use a sterilized spring needle for blood letting or a three-edged needle to prick 0. 2 - 0. 3 cm deep at each point and for letting out 6 - 7 drips of blood, once a day or once every other day, ten days being a course of treatment.

7. Acupoint cutting therapy

Select points on both sides of the 3rd, 4th and 5th

每次任选一对腧穴,每穴注射利血平
0.1～0.2 ml。

（3）方3：足三里、内关、合谷、三
阴交。每次上下肢各取一穴,各穴轮
流使用,每穴注射 0.25% 普鲁卡因
1 ml,每日 1 次,10～15 日次为 1 个
疗程。

6. 刺血疗法

主穴用头维。眩晕,兼前额闷胀
不适者加攒竹;胸闷痛甚者加印堂、
上星;眩晕头额顶痛加百会,剧痛者
再加四神聪;眩晕伴颈项强者加风
池;眩晕欲仆者加太阳穴。用消毒弹
簧刺血针或三棱针,点刺各穴约
0.2～0.3 cm 深,每穴出血 6～7 滴,
每日或隔日 1 次,10 次为 1 个疗程。

7. 穴位割治疗法

取 3、4、5 等胸椎两旁夹脊穴和

高血压病的中医特色疗法

thoracic vertebrae and Xinshu (BL15), Feishu (BL13), Jueyinshu (BL14), Tianzong (SI11) and Jianyu (LI15). After routine sterilization, give each point an intracutaneous injection of 0.1 ml of 2% procaine, then with the needle tip, prick the skin 0.2 cm deep, penetrate horizontally 0.5 cm, and outward through the skin. Then use scalpel to cut up the skin along the needle and cover the non-sutured wound with routine treatment. Use ten points each time, once every other day. The points are used in turn, and four times is a course of treatment. The interval between the courses of treatment is 10 – 30 days.

8. Ear points pressure therapy

Main points: Point for Lowering Blood Pressure, Sympathetic Nerve, Ear-Shenmen, Heart, Groove for Lowering Blood Pressure. Auxiliary points: Kidney, Occiput, and Ear Apex. Stick vaccaria seeds with adhesive plaster to the above points. Apply the main points each time and modify the auxiliary points according to individual cases. Renew the vaccaria seeds every other day, twelve times being a course of treatment.

Section Four   Massage Therapy

According to the clinical reports, among the hypertensives who receive massage therapy to lower high blood pressure, the overwhelming majority are elderly patients

心俞、肺俞、厥阴俞、天宗、肩髃。常规消毒后,每穴皮内注射 2% 普鲁卡因 0.1 ml,用针头刺入皮肤 0.2 cm 转向上沿皮刺入 0.5 cm,再将针尖刺向皮外,挑起皮肤,用手术刀沿针割开,不缝合,常规包扎,每次 10 个穴位,隔日 1 次,穴位轮换选用,4 次为 1 个疗程,每疗程间隔 10～30 日。

8. 耳穴压迫法

主穴选降压点、交感、神门、心、降压沟。配穴选肾、枕、耳尖。将王不留行子分别用胶布贴于上穴,主穴必贴,配穴随证加减,每 2 日换新子 1 次,12 次为 1 个疗程。

(四)推拿疗法

临床报道采用按摩降压法治疗高血压病患者,其中绝大多数是老年久病不愈,常服中西药均无效者,施

高血压病的中医特色疗法

51

with prolonged hypertension, who have tried either western medicines or Chinese herbal medicines with no effects. The head (forehead, vertex and occiput), the waist and the back, the chest, and the four limbs are usually the regions for massage. After two months' treatment, the high blood pressure is lowered by an average of 8.66 −4.67 kPa. Besides, walking or standing with massage shoes on for 30 minutes respectively in the morning and in the evening also helps to reduce high blood pressure.

Section Five   Physical Exercise Therapy

Though clinical experiment can not as yet prove that physical exercise can evidently lower high blood pressure, regular physical training can improve one's health effectively and reduce or prevent the occurrence of disease. Therefore, regularly performing exercises such as running, quick walking, cycling and swimming are good for those who suffer from mild hypertension. Mental health and relaxation brought about by regular exercises can beneficially affect human body. In traditional Chinese medicine, there has been rich experience in health-care exercise. For instance, taijiquan, eight-diagram brocade (a maneuver in dynamic qigong), yijinjing (limbering-up exercises for the tendons), five-animal boxing, etc. are

术部位为头部(前额、头顶、枕部)、腰背部、胸部及四肢部,经治疗两个月后,血压平均下降 $8.66 \sim 4.67$ kPa。另外,每日早晚各穿按摩鞋(上面有长短细齿,可刺激足底穴位),站立或走动 30 分钟,也有降压作用。

(五)体育疗法

临床试验尚未能证实运动能引起血压明显的下降。但经常锻炼身体,能增强体质,减少或防止疾病的发生。故有规则的体育运动(如跑步、快走、骑自行车、游泳等)对轻型高血压病患者是有益的,规则运动引起的精神上健康和放松对机体会产生有利影响。传统中医学在保健体育方面积累了丰富的经验,如太极拳、八段锦、易筋经、五禽戏等,都是行之有效的防病治病措施。

高血压病的中医特色疗法

all very effective measures for preventing and curing diseases.

But the patients with severe or moderate hypertension should avoid competitive sports, especially the sports for building up muscles (such as weight lifting, gripping, weight holding). If a hypertensive takes excessive exercises, sudden death related to exercise may happen to him. Therefore, the hypertensives with cardiovascular risk factors should be more careful, especially when they have the symptoms as dyspnea and chest pain while doing exercise. It is better to do some tests before taking part in physical exercises so as to decide on proper amount and time for exercise.

Hypertensives who take part in physical training should be cautious of choosing medicines for lowering high blood pressure. It is inadvisable for the patients who maintain large amount of exercise to take Beta-blockers and it is advisable for the hypertensives who take part in short-term exercises to take diuretic to reduce the plasma volume when they are taking exercises.

The amount of exercise depends on heart rate and there is Karvonen formula for calculating it.

Heart rate while exercising = $[X \cdot (\text{maximum heart rate} - \text{heart rate while resting})] + \text{heart rate while resting}$.

但中、重型高血压病患者应避免竞赛性运动,尤其是锻炼肌肉的运动(如举重、握力和持重物)。高血压病患者如运动不适量,可能发生与运动有关的猝死,故合并其他心血管病危险因素者,特别是患者出现运动时呼吸困难或胸痛症状时,更应注意。运动训练前最好作运动试验,以选择合适的运动强度及时间。

参加运动训练的高血压病患者选用降压药物应慎重,维持较大运动量的患者不宜服用β阻滞剂,参加短期训练的高血压病患者用利尿剂可减少血浆容量。

训练的强度依心率而定,可根据Karvonen公式计算训练强度。

运动时心率=[X·(最大心率-休息时心率)]+休息时心率

Small amount of exercise: $X < 50\%$

Moderate amount of exercise: $X = 50\% - 75\%$

Large amount of exercise: $X > 75\%$

Maximum heart rate can be either estimated by exercise test or calculated with the formula: maximum heart rate = 210 − age. This formula is not very accurate, for it is sometimes influenced by anti-hypertensive drugs. As for an individual, one should start with exercise of moderate amount and gradually increase the amount of exercise. This is because most of the hypertensives are middle-aged and elderly people and they used not to have much exercise, so they should increase the amount of exercise step by step.

Section Six   Mental Therapy

Traditional Chinese medical theory holds that mental activity has close relations with human being's physiological and pathological changes. A happy and relaxed mind leads to harmonious balance of qi and blood and fluency of qi movement, resulting in normal functional activities of zang-fu organs and good health. Conversely, sudden or repeated, continual emotional frustrations may result in disorder in functional activities of qi and incoordination between qi and blood, between yin and yang, and

X<50%为轻度运动量

X=50%～75%为中度运动量

X>75%为重度运动量

最大心率可用运动试验估计,也可用公式:最大心率=210－年龄计算。该公式并非十分精确,有时受降压药物作用影响。对个体来说,先从轻度或中强度的运动开始,逐步加大运动量。而大多数高血压病患者是中、老年人,过去没有经常运动的习惯,因此要循序渐进。

(六)情志疗法

中医理论认为精神情志活动,与人的生理病理变化有着密切的关系。心情舒畅,精神愉快则机体气血和调,气机调畅,功能活动正常,身体健康。反之,突然的精神刺激,或反复、持续的精神刺激,可使人体气机逆乱,气血阴阳失调而发病。传统中医学的这种认识与西方医学的理论是一致的。在高血压病的发病因素中,

thus causing diseases. This knowledge in traditional Chinese medicine is in accord with the related theory in western medicine. And this is what is described in the mental source theory and is considered as one of the factors causing hypertension. It is reported that the incidence of hypertension in those who are mentally injured or hot-tempered is evidently higher than that in normal people. This is undoubtedly the theoretical basis of the prevention of hypertension. Therefore, from the angle of prevention, it is advisable for people to be open-minded, avoid harmful irritation and get rid of distracting thoughts, thus keeping in a tranquil mood and getting healthy qi. As a result, hypertension will not occur.

Section Seven   Dietotherapy

Dietotherapy, long ago recorded in Chinese medical works, is widely spread in China. Practitioners of Chinese medicine in ancient and modern times have all attached great importance to the effect of dietotherapy, hence there is a saying: " dietotherapy is better than medication". The dietotherapy of traditional Chinese medicine is simple, convenient and inexpensive. Those foods which are easy to prepare, inexpensive in price and effective for lowering blood pressure are usually the choices for the prevention and treatment of hyperten-

精神源学说所描述的就是这个道理。有报道指出，人群中有精神创伤或性格急躁者，其高血压病患病率明显高于正常人群，这无疑是这种预防理论的一个实践结果。因此，从预防的角度讲，人要做到心情开朗，避免不良的精神刺激，不要有过多的杂念，这样便能"恬淡虚无，真气从之"，高血压病也就不会发生了。

（七）饮食疗法

饮食疗法在中医学中早有记载。饮食疗法（简称食疗）应用颇为广泛，古今中医临床医师都非常重视食疗的作用，故有"药治不如食疗"的说法。中医的食疗具有简、便、廉的特点，可适当选用一些食用方便、价格低廉但又确有降压作用的食物，以达到防治高血压病的目的。具有降压作用或对高血压病患者的症状有治疗作用的食物，约有如下数种，医师

sion. As medicine and food are of the same origin, most of these foods are actually edible medicines, therefore, it is obvious that there is the material base for bringing down blood pressure. The following are the foods which have the effect on bringing down high blood pressure or the curative effect on the symptoms of the hypertensives. But guidance should be given to the hypertensives in selecting and using these foods according to individual cases.

1. Shepherd's purse

Shepherd's purse is an edible wild herb, whose spears are picked and cooked for food in early spring, pleasant and tasty. It contains vitamin B, vitamin C, carotene, niacin, flavone glucoside, potassium bursinate, choline, acetyl choline, etc. Experiments on animals show that shepherd's purse really has an antihypertensive effect. Clinically, to treat hypertension and fundus hemorrhage, decoct 15 g of the flower of shepherd's purse together with 12 g of Mohanlian, take this decoction three times a day, fifteen days in succession being a course of treatment. In the meantime, measure the patient's blood pressure. If the blood pressure is not reduced, continue to take the decoction for another course of treatment. When the blood pressure is obviously reduced, take the decoction twice a day and properly reduce the dosage.

可根据高血压病患者的具体情况,指导其酌情选用。

1. 荠菜

荠菜,又名荠,初春采其嫩苗作野菜食用清香可口。全草富含维生素 B 类及维生素 C、胡萝卜素、烟酸、黄酮苷、荠菜酸钾、胆碱、乙酰胆碱及干酸胺等。动物实验表明,本品确有降压之功用。临床上,凡高血压、眼底出血,用荠菜花15 g,墨旱莲12 g,水煎服,每日 3 次,连服 15 日为 1 个疗程,同时监测血压水平;如血压未降可继续服用 1 个疗程;若血压已明显降低,可酌减,每日 2 次,每次量略为减少。

2. Spinage

Containing protein, fat, carbohydrate, coarse fiber, calcium, phosphorus, iron, carotene, nicotinic acid, vitamin C, oxalic acid, etc., spinage can promote blood circulation and functional activities of five zang-organs, lower the adverse qi and regulate middle energizer, it can also slake thirst and moisturize the intestines; applicable to hypertension and chronic constipation. For the hypertensives manifested as constipation, headache, flushed complexion and dizziness, steep fresh spinage in boiling water for 3 minutes, then mix it with sesame oil to make it ready to eat. Take 250 –300 g of it every day in two doses, ten days being a course of treatment. It can be taken continuously.

3. Malan

Malan is also called Lubianju in Chinese. Usually its tender rhizome which is called Malantou, is picked and cooked for food in spring. It contains protein, vitamin C, organic acid, etc. For the patients with hypertension, fundus hemorrhage or feeling of distending pain in the eyeball, decoct 30 g of Malantou together with 15 g of Shengdihuang with water and take the decoction twice a day, ten days being a course of treatment. If there is no side effect, it can be taken continuously for a period so as to observe its effects.

2. 菠菜

内含蛋白质、脂肪、碳水化合物、粗纤维、钙、磷、铁、胡萝卜素、尼克酸、维生素C、草酸等。能利五脏,通血脉,下气调中,止渴,润肠。适用于高血压、慢性便秘。高血压病患者便秘、头痛、面赤、目眩,可用新鲜菠菜置沸水中烫约3分钟,以麻油拌食,每日2次,日食250～300 g,每10日为1个疗程。可以连续食用。

3. 马兰

又称路边菊,春天采其嫩茎(马兰头)做菜吃。马兰头含蛋白质、维生素C、有机酸等。高血压、眼底出血、眼球胀痛,用马兰头30 g,生地黄15 g,煎水服,每日2次,10日为1个疗程。如无不适等副作用出现,可持续服用一个时期,以观后效。

4. Pea plant

The sprouts of pea plant can be cooked for food. Its seeds are edible and can be ground into flour for preparing food. For hypertensives, get an appropriate amount of pea sprouts, wash it and pound it into pulp. Then use a piece of sanitary gauze to squeeze juice from it. Warm the juice and take half a cup of it each time, twice a day, ten days being a course of treatment.

5. Jew's ear

Jew's ear has the functions of nourishing the stomach, supplementing qi, cooling blood, reducing blood pressure, promoting diuresis and strengthening the body. For the patient with hypertension, angiosclerosis and fundus hemorrhage, soak 30 g of Jew's ear in water for one night, steam it for 1 - 2 hours, add some crystal sugar and take it before going to bed. Take it once a day and ten days is a course of treatment. It can be taken continuously since it has no side effect.

6. Watermelon

Watermelon has the functions of removing summer heat, quenching thirst, and promoting diuresis, applicable to hypertension, nephritis, coronary heart disease, etc. For the hypertensives, decoct 10 g of watermelon pericarp together with 10 g of Caojueming, drink the decoction several times a day as a substitute of tea, ten days

4. 豌豆

嫩苗色青,摘其梢头,可做蔬菜,种子可食,磨成粉可做面。高血压病患者,取豌豆苗1把,洗净捣烂,用卫生纱布包榨汁饮,每次半茶杯,略加温服。每日2次,10日为1个疗程。

5. 木耳

本品能滋胃益气、凉血、降压利便、滋补强壮。凡高血压、血管硬化、眼底出血者,可用本品30 g,清水浸泡一夜,于锅上蒸1～2小时,加入适量冰糖,于睡前服用,每日1次,10日为1个疗程,可持续服用,无任何副作用。

6. 西瓜

西瓜具有消暑、解渴、利尿的功效。适用于高血压、肾炎、冠心病等。高血压病患者,取西瓜翠衣10 g,草决明10 g,煎汤代茶,口服数次,10日为1个疗程,长服更为有利。另外,凡心血管病患者,在西瓜应市期间,最好

高血压病的中医特色疗法

being a course of treatment. It would be more beneficial to take this decoction for a long period. Besides, it is better for the patients with cardiovascular disease to have watermelon every day when it is in season. Continual intake of watermelon instead of drinking tea, especially in hot days, will inevitably contribute to curative effect.

7. Persimmon

It is proved by experiment data that tannin in persimmon juice and flavone glucoside extracted from persimmon leaf can lower blood pressure and increase the blood flow of the coronary artery, hence it is beneficial to the functional activity of the heart. Persimmon is a good medicine for lowering blood pressure and markedly effective for preventing and curing hypertension, cardiovascular disease, constipation and piles. For the patients suffering from hypertension or coronary heart disease, mix wild persimmon juice with milk or rice water and add proper amount of crystal sugar, take half a cup of this mixture each time as a measure to prevent and cure paralytic stroke. In daily life, the dried persimmon is used to cook with proper amount of water until it is tender enough and taken as a usual dessert. Take 50–80 g each time, twice a day.

8. Apple

The modern medical research has proved that apple

每日食之,尤其在夏天炎热之际,可
以西瓜代茶,持续食用。

7. 柿子

据实验资料证实,柿汁含单宁成
分、柿叶中提取的黄酮甙能降低血
压,并能增加冠状动脉的血流量。柿
子为降压良药,对于防治高血压病、
心血管病及便秘、痔疾有显效。高血
压病、冠心病患者,取野生柿榨汁,以
牛奶或米汤调服,可酌加适量冰糖,
每服半茶杯,可用以预防中风。平时
可取柿饼适量加水煮烂,当点心吃,
每日 2 次,每次 50~80 g,常服有效。

8. 苹果

现代医学研究结果证明,苹果能

can prevent the increase of cholesterol in the blood. It is advisable for patients with hypertension or coronary heart disease to take apples constantly all the year round, at least one or two apples a day.

9. Garlic

Garlic contains garlic glucoside, which has the function of reducing blood pressure. Take 1 – 2 heads of sugar-vinegar garlic every morning on empty stomach and at the same time drink some sugared vinegar in which the garlic is soaked. Take this continually for half a month, and the blood pressure will be brought down.

10. Other foods effective for lowering blood pressure

(1) Penghaocai: Rinse and mash the fresh Penghaocai, mix it with warm water and drink a small cup of it twice a day.

(2) Carrot: Rinse and liquidize the carrot for drinking.

(3) Sweet potato: Peel it and crush it into pulp. Mix it with cool boiled water and drink a small cup of it, 2 – 3 times a day, which is also effective for relaxing the bowels.

(4) Wild rice shoot and celery: Decoct 30 – 60 g of wild rice shoot and 30 g of celery with water and take the decoction, which can also cure constipation.

(5) Yulanhua: Take 3 – 6 g a day. Pour boiling water on it and drink it as the substitute of tea, or decoct 12 – 18 g

防止血胆固醇的增高。高血压病、冠心病患者宜四季不间断食用苹果,至少每天吃 1～2 个。

9. 大蒜

大蒜含大蒜甙,有降压作用。每天早晨空腹吃糖醋大蒜 1～2 个,并可同时喝一些浸大蒜的糖醋液汁,连服半个月,可使血压下降。

10. 其他有效降压食物

(1) 蓬蒿菜:新鲜蓬蒿菜洗净后,切细捣汁,温开水和服,每次 1 小杯,日服 2 次。

(2) 胡萝卜:洗净后捣汁服用。

(3) 地瓜:去皮捣烂绞汁,凉开水和服,每次 1 小杯,日服 2～3 次,并有通便作用。

(4) 茭白、芹菜:鲜茭白 30～60 g,芹菜 30 g,加水煎服,并可治疗便秘。

(5) 玉兰花:每日 3～6 g,沸水冲泡代茶,或鲜叶 12～18 g,加水

of the fresh leaves with water and take the decoction.

(6) Tomato: Take 1 – 2 fresh tomatoes on empty stomach every morning.

(7) Eggplant: The purple eggplant contains vitamin P. Taking it over a long period of time will help prevent and cure hypertension.

(8) Mungbean: Mungbean has the function of clearing away heat and promoting diuresis. So it is good for hypertensives with heat-syndrome and signs of edema.

(9) Corn and corn silk: Corn and corn silk have the function of promoting diuresis and reducing blood pressure. Clinically, they are used to cure hypertension and edema caused by nephritis. Decoct 30 g of corn silk, 30 g of banana peel and 10 g of Zhizi with water. This decoction is applicable to the hypertensives with hemorrhinia.

(10) Lotus and lotus root: Lotus and lotus root can cure hypertension and the complications of feeling of fullness in the head, palpitation and insomnia. Add boiling water to 1.5 g of lotus plumule and drink it as the substitute of tea. Decoct 3 – 4 nodes of lotus root and take the decoction.

(11) Haw: Decoct 10 –20 g of haw or 3 –10 g of haw flower with water and take the decoction.

(12) Sesame: Decoct 30 g of sesame stem together with 15 g of Xixiancao and 15 g of Chouwutong with

煎服。

（6）番茄：鲜番茄 1～2 只，每日早晨空腹吃。

（7）茄子：紫茄中含维生素 P，久服对防治高血压病有利。

（8）绿豆：具有清热利水作用，高血压病患者伴有热象或浮肿倾向者颇宜。

（9）玉米、玉米须：有较明显的利尿及降压作用。临床上常用来治疗肾炎引起的浮肿和高血压病。玉米须、香蕉皮各30 g，栀子10 g，加水煎服，可治高血压病患者的鼻衄。

（10）莲、藕：可治高血压病伴头胀、心悸、失眠。莲子心1.5 g，可沸水冲泡代茶饮。藕节 3～4 个，可加水煎服。

（11）山楂：山楂 10～20 g 或山楂花 3～10 g，加水煎服。

（12）芝麻：芝麻梗30 g，与豨莶草、臭梧桐各15 g，加水煎服，可治高

water. This decoction is effective for hemiplegia caused by hypertensive apoplexy.

(13) Calabash: Crush the fresh calabash into pulp and squeeze it for juice. Then mix the juice with honey. Take one small cup of it a time, twice a day.

(14) Banana: Decoct 30 – 60 g of banana peel or banana stalk with water, or decoct the banana flower. These decoctions are applicable to the prevention of apoplexy.

(15) Pear: Pear has the functions of lowering blood pressure, clearing away heat and tranquilizing the mind. It is effective for the hypertensives with dizziness, palpitation and tinnitus.

(16) Tangerine and tangerine pith: Tangerine and tangerine pith contain vitamin P. It is effective for the hypertensives to take them over a long period of time.

(17) Preserved egg: Eat 2 – 3 preserved eggs dipped in some sugared vinegar every day.

(18) Dried mussel meat: Grind it into powder. Eat a preserved egg with this powder once every evening.

(19) Dried sea cucumber: Cook 60 – 90 g of sea cucumber with appropriate amount of crystal sugar until it is tender. Eat it every day on empty stomach.

(20) Dried jellyfish: Rinse 60 – 90 g of dried jellyfish so as to get rid of its saline taste. Boil it with equal

血压中风后半身不遂。

(13)葫芦:鲜葫芦捣烂取汁,以蜂蜜调服,每次1小杯,口服2次。

(14)香蕉:香蕉皮或柄30~60 g,煎汤口服。香蕉花加水煎服,能预防中风。

(15)梨:具有降压、清热及镇静作用,高血压病症见头晕目眩,心悸耳鸣者颇适宜。

(16)橘及橘络:含维生素 P,久服对高血压病患者有利。

(17)皮蛋:每日2~3只,用糖醋蘸食。

(18)淡菜:15 g,干燥后研细末,用皮蛋1只蘸细末,每晚食1次。

(19)海参:30 g,加适量冰糖煮烂,每日空腹服用。

(20)海蜇:60~90 g,漂洗去除咸味,同荸荠等量煮汤服用。适用于

amount of water chestnut and take the decoction, which is applicable to hypertension with hyperactive liver-yang accompanied with hyperlipemia.

(21) Vinegar-prepared peanuts: Soak proper amount of peanuts in edible vinegar for 7 days. Eat 10 peanuts both in the morning and in the evening, which can help lower blood pressure.

Chapter Two   Treatment for Senile Primary Hypertension

Hypertension is a disease commonly seen in the elderly. From the 1979 – 1980 nationwide investigation of hypertension, the morbidity rate is 35% in persons aged 65 and older, 5% between 35 to 45 years. Unlike the young, the elderly case is characterized by elevated systolic pressure, but with normal or relatively lower diastolic pressure. As a risk factor of cardiovascular and cerebrovascular diseases, elevation of systolic pressure is more critical than that of diastolic pressure or of mean pressure. Senile hypertension thus has its own characteristics in pathogenesis, clinical manifestation, treatment and prognosis.

Senile hypertension may not be noticed, since it sometimes has no obvious symptoms and can be neglected

Typical TCM Therapy for Primary Hypertension

肝阳上亢型高血压伴高脂血症者。

（21）醋泡花生：花生米适量，加食醋浸泡 7 日，每日早晚吃花生米 10 粒，有助降压。

二、老年高血压病的治疗

高血压病是老年人的常见病。据 1979～1980 年全国高血压普查资料，65 岁以上高血压病患病率约为 35％，而 35～45 岁组则为 5％。与较年轻者不同，老年人高血压病是以收缩压升高为主，舒张压往往不高或相对偏低。作为心脑血管疾病的危险因素，单独收缩压升高要比舒张压或平均压升高更为重要。所以，老年人高血压病在发病机理、临床表现、治疗及预后等方面均有其特殊性。

老年性高血压病无典型症状者较多，易被忽略或被其他疾病所掩

高血压病的中医特色疗法

or concealed by its various complications. According to the investigation, 40%–45% of the elderly aged 60 and older suffer from hypertension. The risk of morbidity of cardiovascular and cerebrovascular among them is eight times higher than that among the healthy.

Some cases of senile hypertension previously suffered from presenile elevated systolic pressure, but in most cases, it develops from the decreased elasticity and compliance of arteries, which result from hyperplasia of endangium and media and from increased contents of collagen, elastose, lipid and calcium. These decrease the dilatancy of big arteries in systolic period, resulting in high systolic pressure, but the intra-arterial pressure can not be maintained in diastolic period, so that the diastolic pressure may reduce and the pulse pressure increases.

In the elderly, hyaline degeneration exists in the arteriolar wall and gradually increases vascular resistance, but cardiac output remains normal or lower. Heart failure may happen, when myocardial hypertrophy and systole and diastole dysfunction becomes obvious.

Hypotensor is used to maintain blood pressure at a normal level, to lessen the damage of the heart, brain and kidney caused by elevated blood pressure, and minimize the risk of hypertensive crisis and other complications. It is very important to take the drugs regularly.

盖,同时合并症较多。据调查,在 60
岁以上的老人中,约 40%～45%患有
高血压病。他们发生心脑血管意外
的危险性比血压正常者高 8 倍。

老年人高血压病,除一部分是从
老年前期的舒张期高血压演变而来
外,大部分是由于血管内膜和中层变
厚,胶原蛋白、弹性蛋白、脂质和钙含
量增加导致大动脉弹性减退,顺应性
下降而产生。这些改变,使收缩期射
血时由于大动脉扩张性降低,收缩压
可以增高。舒张期时则又不能保持
血管腔内压力,故舒张压可以减低,
脉压增大。

老年人中、小动脉壁可发生透明
样变化,逐渐引起血管阻力增大,而
心排血量正常或降低。若心肌肥厚
以及心脏收缩与舒张功能受损比较
明显,则易诱发心力衰竭。

服用降压药的目的主要是维持
血压在正常水平,从而降低高血压对
心、脑、肾等器官损伤,同时也减少了
高血压危象和并发症的发生。因此,
及时服药,按时服药非常重要。但是

高血压病的中医特色疗法

Due to their worries about the side effects or impatience to take the drugs, some patients do not hold on the treatment. The irregular use results in not only drug resistance but also relapse or aggravation and in some serious cases even hypertensive crisis. Therefore the elderly patients should appropriately take hypotensors as follows. Firstly, under the doctor's guidance, take the routine drugs with proper dosage and do not worry about the side effects. If the indications of drugs are fully understood, they could be used properly, safely and effectively. Secondly, drugs used should be as less as possible and mutually compatible, so as to improve curative effects and reduce side effects. Thirdly, drugs with probable side effects on elderly patients should be used with caution. If used, the administration of drugs should be based on the monitoring of blood concentration and of clinical effects. Fourthly, the elderly should not use hypotensor without the doctor's advice. Lastly, administration of drugs for the elderly patients should start with only one kind of drug and in smaller dosage. Usually half dosage is tried at first and then adjustment is made according to the responses of blood pressure and reaction of the body. In the treatment, attention should be paid to the changes of the disease, in order to determine whether the treatment is suitable to the individual condition. Clinical practice has

有不少老年人过分顾虑降压药的副作用,或嫌服药麻烦而服服停停,不能坚持用药。这样一方面易出现"反跳"现象,使血压回升,严重者可发生高血压危象;另一方面,由于血压反复回升将会加重病情,并可能产生耐药性而影响治疗效果。老年人要坚持合理服用降压药,其一,在医生指导下,应用正常的临床治疗药物和剂量,不必顾虑降压药的副作用,掌握好用药指征,不滥用,不乱用,以提高药物治疗的合理性、安全性和有效性。其二,遵循少而精的原则,尽量减少用药种类并注意正确的配伍,以提高药物的疗效,减少药物的不良反应。其三,尽量少用或慎用易使老年人产生不良反应的药物,一旦使用,最好采用血浓度监测与临床疗效观察相结合的方法设计全体化给药方案。其四,引导老年病人不要随意自行应用各种降压药物。其五,对老年人的用药宜从小剂量及单一种类药用起,通常先试用一半剂量,再根据血压及机体反应决定增减。治疗中应仔细观察病情变化,以了解治疗是否

高血压病的中医特色疗法

showed that Chinese herbal medicine is especially suitable for the elderly hypertensive patients. Pathological change in these cases is mainly characterized by yang hyperactivity and yin deficiency associated with blood-stasis and phlegm-dampness. As the disease progresses, deficient yin impairs yang and results in deficiency of both yin and yang. Its basic therapeutic principle hence is to nourish the liver and kidney, regulate yin and yang, promote blood circulation to remove blood-stasis, and resolve phlegm and eliminate dampness. For the cases with yang hyperactivity and yin deficiency, use modified Qiju Dihuang Tang (decoction) and Tianma Gouteng Tang (decoction); for deficiency of yin and yang, use modified Erxian Tang (decoction) and Shenqi Pill; for hyperactivity of liver-fire, use Longdan Xiegan Tang (decoction) with addition of Gouteng and Huaihua; for excessive phlegm-dampness, use Banxia Baizhu Tianma Tang (decoction) with Shichangpu and Zhinanxing added; for internal obstruction of blood-stasis, use modified Taohong Siwu Tang (decoction).

For elderly hypertensives, attention should be paid to non-drug therapy and self health-care. In order to improve the drug effect, stabilize blood pressure and prevent possible accident, it is advisable for them to practice six "dos" and thirteen "don'ts" in daily life.

适合患者的机体状况。大量临床经验表明,中医药尤其适用于老年人高血压病。老年人高血压病多为阴虚阳亢,兼有瘀血、痰湿,随着病情进展,阴损及阳,出现阴阳两虚。所以本病的基本治法是培补肝肾,调和阴阳,活血化瘀,化痰除湿。临床辨证属阴虚阳亢的可用杞菊地黄汤合天麻钩藤饮加减,阴阳两虚型可用二仙汤合肾气丸加减,肝火亢盛型可用龙胆泻肝汤加钩藤、槐花,痰湿壅盛型可用半夏白术天麻汤加石菖蒲、制南星,瘀血内阻型可用桃红四物汤加减。

对于老年高血压病应特别重视非药物治疗,加强自我保健意识,如能做到以下的"六要"、"十三不要",则能加强药物疗效,稳定血压和防止意外。

高血压病的中医特色疗法

Section One   Six "Dos"

1. Prevent and treat hypertension for lifetime and most important of all measure blood pressure regularly. Maintain long-term and proper treatment guided by the doctor and take the drugs regularly and continually.

2. Have a balanced diet. The diet should be on the principle of the "four lows" (low salt, low carbohydrate, low fat and low calorie) and the "three highs" (high vitamin, high calcium and high cellulose).

3. Take part in physical exercises, especially those within their capacity according to individual cases. For instance, walking, Taijiquan, etc., which are helpful to improving the body condition and reducing blood pressure.

4. Keep mental health. Hypertension is a psychosomatic disease, which should be dealt with by the combination of psychotherapy and somatotherapy. Mental stress may promote peripheral nerve to excrete catecholamine, leading to the increase of blood pressure, acceleration of platelet aggregation and even occurrence of apoplexia. Hence, it is very important to keep mental relaxation.

5. Avoid possible accidents. Marked elevation of

（一）六要

1. 要终身防治高血压。最重要的是定期测量血压，做到心中有数。要在医师的指导下坚持长期合理的治疗，坚持服药。

2. 要合理营养，平衡膳食。应遵循"四低"（低盐、低糖、低脂、低热量）和"三高"（高维生素、高钙和平衡蛋白质、高纤维素）原则，调整饮食结构，节制饮食。

3. 要积极运动。多参加适合个体的、力所能及的活动，如散步、打太极拳等，对改善症状、降低血压有益。

4. 要保持心理健康。高血压病是一种"心身疾病"，故须采取心理治疗和躯体治疗相结合的办法。精神紧张可使神经末梢纤维分泌的儿茶酚胺增加，使血压升高，还可激发血小板的凝聚作用，甚至导致脑血管意外的发生。因此，放松精神，保持健康的心理十分重要。

5. 要避免随机事故，如跌倒、过

blood pressure may be caused by tumbling, crouching, laughing and choking, etc. and it may further result in accidents.

6. Be alert to apoplexy aura. Apoplexy is most likely caused by hypertension, and the following are the premonitory signs, for instance, sudden loss of vision for several seconds or minutes; temporary blurred vision or visual field defect; dizziness on turning the head, slurred speech, etc.

Section Two   Thirteen "Don'ts"

1. Don't withdraw antihypertensive drugs suddenly. It is necessary to take the drugs continually to maintain normal blood pressure. Withdrawing the drugs without the doctor's permission may result in sudden rise of blood pressure and even an emergency will occur.

2. Don't be in an anxious state of mind. Keep light-hearted and open-minded.

3. Don't be listless. Take proper and regular physical exercises, which is helpful to reducing blood pressure, but strenuous exercise may lead to sudden rise of blood pressure.

4. Don't eat too much. In the elderly, overeating may cause elevation of diaphragm and further weaken

分低头、大笑、憋气等,防止突然诱发血压剧烈升高而导致意外。

6. 要警惕中风先兆。高血压病最易导致脑中风,所以要警惕以下先兆症状,防患于未然,如眼前突然发黑,持续数秒或数分钟;短时间视物模糊或视野缺损;转头时头晕,说话不清等。

(二)十三不要

1. 不要突然停服降压药。高血压病需连续服药方能控制血压在正常水平,若未经医师同意,随意停服降压药,可导致血压陡然升高,产生意外。

2. 不要情绪波动。保持轻松愉快的情绪,心胸豁达,及时排除不良情绪的干扰,这对老年高血压病患者十分重要。

3. 不要身懒。要坚持适当的体育锻炼,这有助于降压,但要注意避免剧烈运动而致血压骤升。

4. 不要饮食过饱。老年人胃肠功能下降,过饱后膈肌上抬,使心肺

gastrointestinal function, which may interfere with the functions of the heart and lung. On the other hand, a large quantity of blood concentrating in the gastrointestinal tract may induce insufficient blood supply of the heart and brain, and the damage of these organs will be aggravated.

5. Don't reduce the sleeping time. Insufficient sleep tends to cause fluctuation of blood pressure. If a hypertensive patient fails to sleep all night, his blood pressure may be elevated by 2.0 -4.0 kPa next morning.

6. Don't be stimulated by cold. Avoid washing hands, feet and face with cold water. Since there are abundant blood vessels in these areas, cold stimulation will cause contraction of the peripheral blood vessels, resulting in elevation of blood pressure.

7. Don't be overstrained. Since overstrain may induce elevation of blood pressure, the elderly patient should pay attention to rest and try to avoid overstrain.

8. Don't defecate with strength. The elderly is liable to habitual constipation. Defecating with excessive strength will increase abdominal pressure and further cause elevation of blood pressure, possibly resulting in cerebral apoplexy or myocardial infarction.

9. Don't suddenly change the posture. Blood reserve in the brain is relatively small in the elderly patient and the regulatory function of the cerebral vessels is weak-

功能受限,加之大量血液集中胃肠道,而致心脑供血不足,加重器官的损害。

5. 不要减少睡眠。睡眠不足易导致血压波动。高血压病患者彻夜失眠,次晨血压可增高 2.0 ～ 4.0 kPa。

6. 不要寒冷刺激。避免用冷水洗手、洗脚、洗脸。因此处的血管和神经分布极为丰富,受冷刺激后导致末梢血管收缩,血压上升。

7. 不要疲劳。疲劳会诱发血压升高,故老年高血压病患者应注意休息,避免疲劳。

8. 不要用力排便。老年人易发生习惯性便秘,若排便进力过度,腹压升高引起血压骤升,可能导致脑中风或心肌梗死。

9. 不要体位突变。老年高血压病患者心脑储备功能较差,脑血管对脑血流量的调节功能减退,当体质突

ened. Therefore, a sudden change of posture, for instance, suddenly standing up after a long-time squatting, may result in faint.

10. Don't watch TV for a long time. Radiation of TV will harm the body, and prolonged TV watching may cause visual tiredness and increase blood pressure.

11. Don't have a "high salt, high carbohydrate, high cholesterol and high calorie" diet. High salt diet may increase blood pressure; high cholesterol can cause hyperlipemia and atherosclerosis; high carbohydrate and high calorie will lead to weight gain and disturbance of carbohydrate metabolism. All these may aggravate the illness.

12. Don't talk too much. It is better for the elderly patient to speak less and listen more. Excessive talking may accelerate catecholamine excretion, leading to faster heart beat, increase of oxygen consumption, and elevation of blood pressure.

13. Don't fasten the collar, shoelace and trousers belt tightly. The tightly fastened collar and tie may stimulate the carotid sinus and increase blood pressure. The tightly fastened trousers belt may obstruct blood circulation below the waist to a certain degree, causing elevation of blood pressure. And the tightly fastened shoelace may increase blood pressure via nerve reflex.

然改变,如久蹲后突然站起,易发生
晕厥。

10. 不要久看电视。看电视久
了,电视辐射对人体有影响,视觉易
疲劳,会导致血压上升。

11. 不要"四高"饮食。"四高"指
高盐、高糖、高胆固醇、高热量饮食。
高盐饮食使血压升高,高胆固醇饮食
易造成高脂血症、动脉粥样硬化,高
糖、高热量饮食使人发胖,体重增加
和糖代谢紊乱,这些均可能会加重高
血压病的病情。

12. 不要多说话。高血压病老人
宜多听少说,因说话过多,体内儿茶
酚胺分泌增多,心跳加快,氧耗增加,
血压升高。

13. 不要扣紧衣领、裤带和鞋带。
若领扣、领带过紧,刺激了颈动脉窦,
而使血压升高。紧勒裤带时,腰以下
部位的血流受到一定阻碍,心脏势必
增加泵血功能而血压升高。鞋带过
紧亦会通过神经反射使血压升高。

高血压病的中医特色疗法

Chapter Three   Treatment for Chief Manifestations of Primary Hypertension

Primary hypertension is a systemic chronic cardiovascular disease, with chief manifestations of headache, dizziness, palpitation and numbness of extremities, etc. It is included in the categories of diseases known as "headache", "dizziness" or "liver-wind" in traditional Chinese medicine, and related to "palpitation", "chest-qi obstruction" and "apoplexy" to a certain degree.

Section One   Headache

1. Hyperactivity of liver-yang

Chief manifestations: Distending or dragging pain of head, dizziness, which is usually induced by mental stress, flushed face, conjunctival congestion, bitter taste in the mouth, tinnitus, reddish tongue and wiry pulse.

Therapeutic principle: Calm the liver and suppress yang.

Prescription: Modified Tianma Gouteng Yin (decoction), composed of Gouteng 12 g (decocted later), Tianma 6 g, Shijueming 25 g (decocted first), Zhenzhumu 25 g (decocted first), Juhua 10 g, Huainiuxi 12 g, Huangqin 10 g, Luobumaye 15 g, Xuanshen 10 g and

三、高血压病主症的治疗

原发性高血压病是一种全身性慢性心血管疾病。主症有头痛、眩晕、心慌、肢麻等。属于中医学"头痛"、"眩晕"、"肝风"等范畴,并与"心悸"、"胸痹"、"中风"等有一定关系。

(一)头痛

1. 肝阳上亢

【证候】 头胀痛或掣痛,目眩,常因精神紧张而诱发,面红目赤,口苦,耳鸣如轰。舌质红,脉弦。

【治法】 平肝潜阳。

【方药】 天麻钩藤饮加减。钩藤(后下)12 g,天麻6 g,石决明(先煎)25 g,珍珠母(先煎)25 g,菊花10 g,怀牛膝12 g,黄芩10 g,罗布麻叶15 g,玄参10 g,白芍药12 g。

Baishaoyao 12 g.

Modification: Add Longgu 15 g (decocted first) and Muli 30 g (decocted first) for hyperactivity of liver-yang with dizziness, flushed face and dry eyes; add Shengdihuang 9 g, Cishi 30 g (decocted first) or Liuwei Dihuang Wan (bolus) 3 g swallowed for deficiency of kidney-yin with sore lumbus and tinnitus.

2. Stirring-up of liver-wind

Chief manifestations: Head dragging pain, dizziness, as if suffering from seasickness, tinnitus, dim eyesight, falling down in a faint, stiffness and spasm of limbs; reddish tongue, wiry pulse.

Therapeutic principle: Calm the liver and suppress wind.

Prescription: Modified Linyang Gouteng Tang (decoction), composed of Gouteng 10 g (decocted later), Juhua 10 g, Baishaoyao 12 g, Guiban 10 g (decocted first), Shengdihuang 12 g, Baijiangcan 10 g, Mudanpi 10 g, Luobumaye 15 g and Linyangjiao 0.3 −0.6 g (swallowed or perfused immediately).

Modification: For delirium, perfuse one pill of Angong Niuhuang Wan (pill).

Section Two   Dizziness

1. Stirring-up of wind-yang

Chief manifestations: Dizziness and dim eyesight, as

【加减】　若眩晕,面红目干,肝阳亢盛者可加龙骨(先煎)15 g,牡蛎(先煎)30 g;若腰酸耳鸣,肾阴不足者可加生地黄9 g,磁石(先煎)30 g,或六味地黄丸3 g吞服。

2. 肝风上扰

【证候】　头部掣痛,眩晕,如坐舟车,耳鸣目花,甚则一时性厥仆,肢体强痉。舌红,脉弦。

【治法】　平肝熄风。

【方药】　羚羊钩藤汤加减。钩藤(后下)10 g,菊花10 g,白芍药12 g,龟版(先煎)10 g,生地黄12 g,白僵蚕10 g,牡丹皮10 g,罗布麻叶15 g,羚羊角(即刻吞服或灌服)0.3～0.6 g。

【加减】　若神昏躁扰不宁者可加安宫牛黄丸1粒(灌服)。

(二)眩晕

1. 风阳上扰

【证候】　眩晕目花,如坐舟车,

if suffering from seasickness; numbness of scalp, or even distending pain; flushed face, irritability, insomnia, dreaminess, conjunctival congestion, bitter taste in the mouth, and accompanied by numbness of lips, tongue and limbs; reddish tongue with thin and yellow coating, wiry and rapid pulse.

Therapeutic principle: Calm the liver and suppress yang, clear away heat and suppress wind.

Prescription: Modified Tianma Gouteng Yin (decoction), composed of Mingtianma 6 g, Gouteng 15 g (decocted later), Shengshijueming 30 g (decocted first), Baijili 10 g, Danhuangqin 10 g, Shengshanzhizi 10 g, Chuanniuxi 12 g, Chuanduzhong 10 g, Mudanpi 10 g and Gandilong 10 g.

Modification: Add Zhenzhumu 30 g (decocted first) for palpitation; add Shenglonggu (decocted first) 30 g, Shengmuli (decocted first) 30 g and Daizheshi 30 g (decocted first) for muscular spasm and tremor.

2. Hyperactivity of yang due to yin deficiency

Chief manifestations: Dizziness, tinnitus, distending pain of head, sore lumbus, weak limbs, amnesia, seminal emission, vexation, dry mouth, insomnia, dreaminess, flushed face; reddish tongue with little coating, wiry, thready and rapid pulse.

Therapeutic principle: Nourish the liver and kidney,

头皮发麻,甚或胀痛,面红烘热,急躁易怒,少寐多梦,目赤口苦,伴唇、舌、肢体麻木。苔薄黄,舌质偏红,脉弦带数。

【治法】 平肝潜阳,清火熄风。

【方药】 天麻钩藤饮加减。明天麻6 g,钩藤(后下)15 g,生石决明(先煎)30 g,白蒺藜10 g,淡黄芩10 g,生山栀子10 g,川牛膝12 g,川杜仲10 g,牡丹皮10 g,干地龙10 g。

【加减】 如有心悸者可加珍珠母(先煎)30 g;如筋惕肉瞤者可加生龙骨(先煎)、生牡蛎(先煎)各30 g,代赭石(先煎)30 g。

2. 阴虚阳亢

【证候】 眩晕耳鸣,头痛头胀,腰酸肢软,健忘遗精,心烦口干,不寐多梦,面红升火。舌质红少苔,脉弦细数。

【治法】 滋补肝肾,平肝潜阳。

calm the liver and suppress yang.

Prescription: Qiju Dihuang Wan with Additions (pill), composed of Gouqizi 12 g, Baijuhua 10 g, Shengdihuang 12 g, Shudihuang 12 g, Shanzhuyu 12 g, Huaishanyao 10 g, Mudanpi 10 g, Fuling 10 g, Zexie 10 g, Tianma 6 g, Gouteng 15 g (decocted later), Shengshijueming 30 g (decocted first), Chuanniuxi 15 g and Zhigancao 5 g.

Modification: Add Zhiguiban 10 g, Nüzhenzi 10 g and Hanliancao 10 g for excessive yin-deficiency; add Chaozhimu 10 g and Huangbo 6 g for pathogenic fire.

Section Three   Palpitation

1. Hyperactivity of fire due to yin deficiency

Chief manifestations: Palpitation, restlessness, insomnia and dizziness, which are aggravated with mental overstrain, feverish sensation in the palms and soles, dreaminess with liability to wake up, tinnitus and sore lumbus; reddish tongue, thready and rapid pulse.

Therapeutic principle: Nourish yin and clear away fire, nourish blood and tranquilize the mind.

Prescription: Modified Tianwang Buxin Dan (pill), composed of Tianmendong 12 g, Maimendong 12 g, Shengdihuang 15 g, Yuzhu 10 g, Danggui 10 g, Huanglian 2 g, Zhizi 6 g, Suanzaoren 12 g, Baiziren 12 g, Fuling 10 g, Fushen 10 g and Danshen 12 g.

【方药】 杞菊地黄丸加味。枸杞子12 g,白菊花10 g,生地黄、熟地黄各12 g,山茱萸12 g,怀山药10 g,牡丹皮10 g,茯苓10 g,泽泻10 g,天麻6 g,钩藤(后下)15 g,生石决明(先煎)30 g,川牛膝15 g,炙甘草5 g。

【加减】 阴虚甚者加炙龟版10 g,女贞子10 g,旱莲草10 g;有火者酌加炒知母10 g,黄柏6 g。

(三)心悸

1. 阴虚火旺

【证候】 心悸,心烦,少寐,头昏,目眩,思虑劳心时加重,手足心热,多梦易醒,耳鸣腰酸。舌质红,脉细数。

【治法】 育阴清火,养血安神。

【方药】 天王补心丹加减。天门冬、麦门冬各12 g,生地黄15 g,玉竹10 g,当归10 g,黄连2 g,栀子6 g,酸枣仁12 g,柏子仁12 g,茯苓、茯神各10 g,丹参12 g。

Modification: For deficiency of kidney-yin, add Zhiguiban 10 g, Shudihuang 12 g, Huangbai 16 g and Zhimu 10 g. For deficiency of liver-yin and stirring-up of deficient wind, manifested as vexation, dizziness and muscular twitching, add Baishaoyao 10 g, Gouqizi 12 g, Zhiheshouwu 10 g, Zhenzhumu 25 g (decocted first) and Muli 25 g (decocted first) to nourish the liver and suppress wind; for deficiency of qi and yin, manifested as shortness of breath and spontaneous perspiration, add Shengmai San (powder).

2. Overabundance of phlegm-fire in the interior

Chief manifestations: Palpitation, insomnia, dreaminess, dizziness, headache, chest distress, epigastric fullness, anorexia and nausea; yellowish and greasy coating, thready and smooth pulse.

Therapeutic principle: Clear away heat and dissipate phlegm.

Prescription: Huanglian Wendan Tang with Additions (decoction), composed of Huanglian 3 g, Fabanxia 10 g, Baizhu 12 g, Tianma 6 g, Fuling 15 g, Chenpi 10 g, Dannanxing 6 g, Shichangpu 10 g, Zhike 10 g and Gancao 6 g.

Section Four   Numbness of Extremities

1. Obstruction of collaterals

Chief manifestations: Consciousness, numbness of

【加减】 肾阴虚加炙龟版10 g,熟地黄12 g,黄柏16 g,知母10 g;肝阴不足,虚风内动,虚烦,头晕,肉𥆧,酌加白芍药10 g,枸杞子12 g,制何首乌10 g,珍珠母(先煎)25 g,牡蛎(先煎)25 g,养肝熄风;气阴两虚,气短自汗,合生脉散。

2. 痰火内盛

【证候】 心悸,少寐,多梦,头晕头痛,胸闷脘胀,食少欲吐。舌苔黄腻,脉细滑。

【治法】 清热化痰。

【方药】 黄连温胆汤加味。黄连3 g,法半夏10 g,白术12 g,天麻6 g,茯苓15 g,陈皮10 g,胆南星6 g,石菖蒲10 g,枳壳10 g,甘草6 g。

(四)肢麻

1. 络脉痹阻

【证候】 神清,肌肤不仁,手足

skin and extremities, stiff tongue, aphasia, or sudden deviation of the eye and mouth, hemiplegia, extremity spasm; reddish tongue with marginal petechia, whitish, thin and greasy coating, wiry and smooth or wiry and thready pulse.

Therapeutic principle: Clear away liver-fire and suppress wind, nourish blood and activate collateral.

Prescription: Modified Tianma Gouteng Yin (decoction), composed of Tianma 10 g, Gouteng 12 g (decocted later), Cijili 10 g, Shijueming 30 g (decocted first), Juhua 6 g, Huangqin 10 g, Fuling 12 g, Huainiuxi 10 g, Danshen 12 g and Sangjisheng 12 g.

Modification: Add Lingyangjiaofen 0.3－0.6 g (swallowed in divided doses) for serious dizziness and headache; add Baishaoyao 10 g and shengdihuang 12 g for yin-deficiency with crimson tongue; add Banxia 10 g, Chenpi 6 g and Zhishi 6 g for abundant expectoration; add Taoren 10 g, Honghua 6 g and Chishaoyao 10 g for purplish tongue with ecchymosis, thready and unsmooth pulse.

2. Blood-stasis due to deficiency of qi

Chief manifestations: Hemiplegia, deviation of the mouth, aphasia, disinclination to speak, numbness of limbs, pale complexion, shortness of breath, lassitude, spontaneous perspiration, palpitation and swelling extremities; darkish pale tongue with thin whitish coating,

麻木,舌强语言不利,或突然口眼㖞斜,半身不遂,或手足拘挛。舌质红,或舌边见瘀点,苔白薄腻,脉弦滑或弦细。

【治法】　清肝熄风,养血通络。

【方药】　天麻钩藤饮加减。天麻10 g,钩藤(后下)12 g,刺蒺藜10 g,石决明(先煎)30 g,菊花6 g,黄芩10 g,茯苓12 g,怀牛膝10 g,丹参12 g,桑寄生12 g。

【加减】　头晕、头痛较甚者加羚羊角粉(分吞)0.3～0.6 g;舌绛红偏阴虚者加白芍药10 g,生地黄12 g;痰多加半夏10 g,陈皮6 g,枳实6 g;舌紫有瘀斑,脉细涩者,酌加桃仁10 g,红花6 g,赤芍药10 g。

2. 气虚血瘀

【证候】　半身不遂,口舌歪斜,言语謇涩或不语,肢体麻木,面色㿠白,气短乏力,自汗心悸,手足肿胀,舌质暗淡,苔薄白,脉细涩无力。

thready and unsmooth pulse.

Therapeutic principle: Replenish qi and nourish blood, promote blood circulation and activate collateral.

Prescription: Modified Buyang Huanwu Tang (decoction), composed of Huangqi 30 g, Taoren 10 g, Honghua 10 g, Chishaoyao 10 g, Dangguiwei 10 g, Chuanxiong 6 g and Dilong 10 g.

Modification: Add Sangpiaoxiao 15 g, Shanzhuyu 12 g, Rougui (decocted later) 5 g and Yizhiren 12 g for aconuresis by astringing and tonifying the kidney; add Chenpi 12 g, Banxia 10 g, Fuling 15 g and Dannanxing 10 g for numbness of limbs to remove wind-phlegm by regulating qi and drying dampness.

Chapter Four   Treatment for Complications of Primary Hypertension

Section One   Hypertensive Encephalopathy

Hypertensive encephalopathy is a series of clinical symptoms, caused by cerebral edema and intracranial hypertension, which results from acute dysfunction of cerebral blood circulation due to persistent cerebral arteriolar spasm in the course of hypertension. It is usually seen in

【治法】 益气养血,活血通络。

【方药】 补阳还五汤加减。黄芪30 g,桃仁10 g,红花10 g,赤芍药10 g,当归尾10 g,川芎6 g,地龙10 g。

【加减】 如小便失禁者,可加桑螵蛸15 g,山茱萸12 g,肉桂(后下)5 g,益智仁12 g等补肾收涩之品;如肢体麻木明显者加陈皮12 g,半夏10 g,茯苓15 g,胆南星10 g,以理气燥湿而祛风痰。

四、高血压病并发症的治疗

(一)高血压脑病

高血压脑病是指在高血压病程中发生脑细小动脉持久性痉挛,导致脑血液循环急性障碍,引起脑水肿和颅内压增高而产生一系列临床症候群,常常好发于急进型或严重缓进型

acute hypertension or serious lingering hypertension with obvious cerebral arteriosclerosis.

1. Diagnostic essentials

(1) Clinical manifestations: a. Usually induced by overstrain, mental stress and emotional agitation. b. Elevation of diastolic pressure, usually DP > 16.0 kPa. c. Symptoms and signs of cerebral edema and intracranial hypertension such as headache, vomiting, restlessness, bradycardia, blurred vision, convulsion, and disturbance of consciousness or even coma. d. Temporary hemiplegia, aphasia and positive pathological nerve reflex. e. Presence of papillary hemorrhage, exudation and edema by fundus examination.

(2) Laboratory examination: Lumbar puncture if necessary. There may be rise of cerebrospinal pressure, and increase of CSF protein content.

2. Characteristics of pathogenesis

In most cases, spleen can be impaired either by irregular diet and especially excessive intake of greasy and sweet food or by anxiety, melancholy and overstrain, resulting in spleen deficiency. Thus the spleen fails to transform and transport dampness, which accumulates and changes into phlegm. In other cases, liver-qi stagnation can cause qi stagnation and dampness accumulation,

高血压伴明显脑动脉硬化的病人。

1. 诊断要点

（1）临床表现：① 本病常因过度劳累、紧张和情绪激动所诱发。② 血压升高以舒张压升高为主，舒张压常超过 16.0 kPa。③ 出现脑水肿和颅内高压的症状，如头痛、呕吐、烦躁不安、心动过缓、视力模糊、抽搐、意识障碍甚至昏迷。④ 可出现暂时性偏瘫、失语、病理性神经反射等征象。⑤ 眼底检查有视神经乳头水肿、渗出、出血。

（2）实验室检查：必要时作脑脊液检查，可有脑脊液压力增高、蛋白含量增高等改变。高血压脑病也有人视为是发生在脑部的高血压危象。

2. 病机特点

本病多因饮食不节，肥甘厚味太过，损伤脾胃，或忧思、劳倦伤脾，以致脾虚，健运失职，水湿内停，湿聚成痰；或肝气郁结，气郁湿滞而生痰。痰阻经络，或兼内生之风火作祟，则表现头痛、眩晕欲仆等症。

which may also change into phlegm. Consequently, phlegm retention in the meridians or production of endogenous fire leads to such symptoms as headache and dizziness.

3. Syndrome differentiation and treatment

(1) Internal excess of phlegm-dampness

Chief manifestations: Dizziness, headache, heaviness of the head, irritability, chest oppression, poor appetite, nausea, sleepiness, fatigue, abdominal distension, pale and enlarged tongue with white and greasy or thick and dry coating, wiry and smooth pulse.

Therapeutic principle: Invigorate the spleen and dissipate dampness, clear away heat and resolve phlegm.

Prescription: Modified Wendan Tang (decoction), composed of Chenpi 10 g, Fabanxia 10 g, Fuling 12 g, Gancao 5 g, Zhike 10 g, Zhuru 10 g, Huanglian 6 g, and Gouteng 15 g (decocted later). Other prescriptions such as Erchen Tang (decoction), Daotan Tang (decoction) and Banxia Baizhu Tianma Tang (decoction) can also be used.

Modification: Add Tianma 9 g, Juhua 10 g and Cijili 12 g for serious dizziness; Cheqianzi 20 g (wrapped) for oliguresis; Yinchen 12 g and Huangqin 10 g for excessive dampness-heat in the liver and gallbladder.

(2) Mental confusion due to turbid-phlegm

Chief manifestations: Serious dizziness, headache,

3. 辨证论治

(1) 痰湿内盛

【证候】 头晕头痛,头重如裹,心烦胸闷,食少欲吐,多眠无力,腹胀痞满。舌胖质淡,苔白腻或厚而无津,脉弦滑。

【治法】 健脾化湿,清热化痰。

【方药】 温胆汤加减。陈皮10 g,法半夏10 g,茯苓12 g,甘草5 g,枳壳10 g,竹茹10 g,黄连6 g,钩藤(后下)15 g。其他可选用二陈汤、导痰汤和半夏白术天麻汤等方治疗。

【加减】 头晕甚者加天麻9 g,菊花10 g,刺蒺藜12 g;尿少加车前子(包煎)20 g;肝胆湿热明显加茵陈12 g,黄芩10 g。

(2) 痰浊蒙闭

【证候】 剧烈头昏,头痛,呕吐,

vomiting, pale complexion, vague mind, aphasia, hemi-plegia, muscular spasm, cool limbs, wheezing sound of sputum in the throat, white and greasy or gray and greasy tongue coating, and sunken and smooth or soft and moderate pulse.

Therapeutic principle: Induce resuscitation with pungent-warm drugs, eliminate phlegm and suppress wind.

Prescription: Modified Ditan Tang (decoction) with Suhexiang Wan (pill), composed of Banxia 10 g, Zhidanxing 10 g, Juhong 6 g, Dangshen 10 g, Fuling 10 g, Gancao 5 g, Zhuru 10 g, Zhishi 10 g, and Shichangpu 10 g, and Suhexiang Wan (pill) 1 - 2 pills (taken separately).

Modification: Add Cangzhu 10 g to expel dampness for excessive phlegm-dampness; add Quanxie 6 g and Wugong 2 pieces for convulsion to suppress wind and stop spasm.

(3) Stagnation of phlegm-heat in the heart

Chief manifestations: Sudden attack of serious headache, followed by frequent vomiting, unconsciousness, wheezing sound of sputum, snore, hemiplegia with limb spasm, convulsion, flushed face, fever, foul breath, irritability, constipation, crimson tongue with yellow, greasy and dry coating, wiry, smooth and rapid pulse.

Therapeutic principle: Clear away heat and resolve

面色苍白,神志昏糊,语言不清,半身不遂,筋脉拘急,四肢不温,痰声辘辘。舌苔白腻或灰腻,脉沉滑或濡缓。

【治法】　辛温开窍,豁痰熄风。

【方药】　涤痰汤合苏合香丸加减。半夏10 g,制胆星10 g,橘红6 g,党参10 g,茯苓10 g,甘草5 g,竹茹10 g,枳实10 g,石菖蒲10 g,苏合香丸(分服)1～2粒。

【加减】　若痰湿重者加苍术10 g以化湿;抽搐加全蝎6 g,蜈蚣2条熄风定搐。

(3)痰热闭窍

【证候】　发病时突然剧烈头痛,随即频繁呕吐,神昏,鼻鼾痰鸣,半身不遂而肢体强痉拘急,面赤身热,口臭,烦躁不宁,大便秘结。舌质红绛,舌苔黄腻而干,脉弦滑数。

【治法】　清热化痰,醒神开窍。

phlegm, induce resuscitation.

Prescription: Lingjiao Gouteng Tang (decoction) with Zhibao Dan (pill) or Angong Niuhuang Wan (pill). The decoction is composed of Lingyangjiao powder 1 g (swallowed in divided doses), Gouteng 10 g (decocted later), Zhenzhumu 0.18 g (infused in divided doses), Shengshijueming 30 g (decocted first), Zhidanxing 10 g, Zhulibanxia 10 g, Tianzhuhuang 10 g, Huanglian 6 g, Shichangpu 10 g, Yujin 6 g, Yuanzhi 10 g, Xiakucao 10 g, and Mudanpi 10 g.

Modification: Add Zhulishui 10 g for abundant sputum to clear away heat and resolve phlegm; add Dahuang (decocted later) 3 -10 g or Mangxiao (infused in divided doses) 5 -10 g for constipation to clear away heat from viscera; add Zhuling 15 g and Cheqianzi 30 g (wrapped) for anuria to promote diureses.

Section Two   Hypertensive Crisis

Hypertensive crisis is a series of clinical symptoms caused by an abrupt rise of blood pressure (especially systolic pressure) due to temporary drastic spasm of systemic arteriolae in the course of hypertension.

1. Diagnostic essentials

(1) Clinical manifestations: a. Usually induced by emotional stress, psychic trauma, tiredness and cold, and

【方药】 羚角钩藤汤合至宝丹或安宫牛黄丸。羚羊角粉(分吞)1 g,钩藤(后下)10 g,珍珠母(分冲)0.18 g,生石决明(先煎)30 g,制胆星10 g,竹沥半夏10 g,天竺黄10 g,黄连6 g,石菖蒲10 g,郁金6 g,远志10 g,夏枯草10 g,牡丹皮10 g。

【加减】 痰多加竹沥水10 g,以清热化痰;大便秘结加生大黄(后下)3～10 g,或芒硝(分冲)5～10 g,以清腑泄热;尿潴留加猪苓15 g,车前子(包煎)30 g以利尿。

(二)高血压危象

高血压危象是指在高血压病程中全身性细小动脉发生暂时性强烈痉挛,导致血压(尤其是收缩压)急剧升高,所引起的一系列临床症候群。

1. 诊断要点

(1)临床表现:① 常因情绪紧张、精神创伤、疲劳、寒冷等诱发,易

mostly seen in lingering hypertension and acute hypertension as well; usually lasting for only a few minutes or a few hours, but occasionally for several days; liable to relapse. b. Elevation of systolic pressure, usually SP > 26.7 kPa. c. Symptoms and signs of vegetative nerve functional disturbance, such as irritability, hyperhidrosis, palpitation, trembling of extremities and pale complexion. d. Angina, heart failure and renal failure.

(2) Laboratory examination: a. Increase of free adrenalin and (or) noradrenalin in serum. b. Increase of blood sugar, a small amount of protein and erythrocyte in urine.

(3) Increase of creatinine, urea nitrogen in serum, and disturbance of water and electrolyte in some cases.

2. Characteristics of pathogenesis

This disease is mostly caused by blockage of blood-stasis in collaterals, and deficiency of yin and yang.

TCM holds that "meridian is involved in new cases and colloateral is invaded in chronic cases", "qi is involved in new cases and blood is affected in chronic cases" and "disorder of qi involves blood and disorder of blood involves qi". Hypertension accelerates arteriolar sclerosis and is complicated with atherosclerosis in many cases. Owing to the disorder of blood vessels and blood circulation, histanoxia, hyperfunction of blood coagulation, etc., blood-stasis symptoms such as unsmooth

发生于缓进型高血压,亦见于急进型高血压,每次发作历时短暂,多为持续几分钟至几小时,偶尔可达数日,且易复发。② 动脉收缩压常超过26.7 kPa。③ 常伴植物神经功能紊乱的症状,如烦躁不安、多汗、心悸、手足发抖、面色苍白等。④ 可伴心绞痛、心力衰竭、肾功能衰竭的症状。

(2) 实验室检查:① 血中游离肾上腺素和(或)去甲肾上腺素增高。② 血糖升高,尿中出现少量蛋白、红细胞等。

(3) 可有血清肌酐、尿素氮升高和水电解质紊乱等。

2. 病机特点

本病多因瘀血阻络,阴阳两虚所致。

中医学认为:"初病在经,久病入络"、"初病在气,久病入血",而"气病则累血,血病则累气"。高血压可促使小动脉硬化,不少合并动脉粥样硬化,由于血液循环、血管功能障碍,组织缺氧及凝血功能的亢进等,临床上可见涩脉、紫绀、淤斑、疼痛等瘀血症状。特别在并发冠状动脉粥样硬化及高血压性心脏病时尤为明显。

pulse, cyanosis, ecchymosis, and pain may be seen, especially in those complicated with coronary heart disease and hypertensive cardiopathy.

In protracted cases, deficient yin may impair yang and consequently cause deficiency of both yin and yang. This pathological change is commonly seen in hypertensives at the late stage and particularly those complicated with coexisting renal failure.

3. Syndrome differentiation and treatment

(1) Blockage of blood-stasis in collaterals

Chief manifestations: Serious headache, dizziness, tinnitus, nausea, vomiting, shortness of breath, stabbing and gripping pain in chest, palpitation, darkish purple complexion and lips, cyanosis of nails, withered and lusterless hair, dark purplish tongue with ecchymosis or hypoglossal varicosity, unsmooth or irregular pulse.

Therapeutic principle: Promote blood circulation to remove blood stasis, activate collaterals and alleviate pain.

Prescription: Modified Xuefu Zhuyu Tang (decoction) and Shixiao San (powder), composed of Taoren 10 g, Honghua 8 g, Danggui 10 g, Shengdihuang 12 g, Chuanxiong 10 g, Huainiuxi 12 g, Zhike 6 g, Yujin 15 g, Danshen 20 g, Wulingzhi 6 g, Puhuang 6 g and Gancao 5 g.

高血压病患者因病久不愈,导致阴损及阳,最终阴阳两虚。这种病机多见高血压病后期患者,尤其是伴有肾脏损害而引起肾功能衰竭者。

3. 辨证论治

（1）瘀血阻络

【证候】　头痛剧烈,头晕耳鸣,恶心呕吐,气急胸痛,如刺如绞,心悸怔忡,面晦唇青,爪甲发绀,毛发干枯。舌质紫暗或见瘀斑,或舌下脉络紫张,脉涩或结代。

【治法】　活血化瘀,通络止痛。

【方药】　血府逐瘀汤合失笑散加减。桃仁10 g,红花8 g,当归10 g,生地黄12 g,川芎10 g,怀牛膝12 g,枳壳6 g,郁金15 g,丹参20 g,五灵脂6 g,蒲黄6 g,甘草5 g。

Modification: Remove Shengdihuang and Niuxi and add Chenxiang 10 g and Tanxiang 10 g for serious pain; add Guizhi 10 g and Xixin 3 g for chilliness and cold limbs.

(2) Deficiency of yin and yang

Chief manifestations: Extreme weakness, intolerance to cold, feverish palms and soles, thirst with little drinking, sore lumbus and knees, loose or dry stool, yellowish-red or copious clear urine, pale and enlarged tongue with teeth marks on the margins, sunken thready or sunken weak pulse.

Therapeutic principle: Warm yang and tonify qi, nourish kidney-yin.

Prescription: Modified Jingui Shenqi Wan (pill), composed of Fuzi 10 g, Rougui (decocted later) 6 g, Shengdihuang 10 g, Shanzhuyu 10 g, Baizhu 10 g, Zexie 15 g, Fuling 30 g, Huainiuxi 10 g and Mudanpi 6 g.

Chapter Five   Regimen for Primary Hypertension

Section One   Body Weight Reduction

Although not all patients with hypertension are overweight, most of the obese persons suffer from hypertension. Since body weight reduction helps to lower obesity,

【加减】 痛剧去生地黄、牛膝，加沉香10 g,檀香10 g;伴恶寒肢冷加桂枝10 g,细辛3 g。

（2）阴阳两虚

【证候】 极度乏力，畏寒肢冷，手足心热，口干欲饮，饮水不多，腰膝酸痛，大便偏溏或干结，小便黄赤或清长。舌质淡胖有齿印，脉象沉细或沉弱。

【治法】 温阳益气，滋补肾阴。

【方药】 金匮肾气丸加减。附子10 g,肉桂（后下）6 g,生地黄10 g,山茱萸10 g,白术10 g,泽泻15 g,茯苓30 g,怀牛膝10 g,牡丹皮6 g。

五、高血压病的摄生调护

（一）减轻体重

并非所有的高血压病患者都是肥胖的，但是，肥胖者中血压升高者居多。对于肥胖的高血压病患者，首

the measure to take first is to reduce body weight for the case with obesity. In overweight patients with mild hypertension, weight reduction may be carried out by reducing calorie intake and increasing physical activity; while in those with moderate and severe hypertension, drugs for lowering blood pressure should be administered at the same time.

Section Two   Limitation of Salt Intake

Limitation of salt intake is one of the methods for hypertension treatment. Modern study shows that intake of sodium chloride less than 400 mg daily is effective for lowering blood pressure. For moderate and severe hypertension, sodium salt intake reduced to 2 g daily together with increased intake of potassium for several months can lower blood pressure to a certain degree. However, it has not been proved effective for the mild case, and only suitable for short-term use.

Section Three   Abstention from Smoking and Limitation of Alcohol Intake

Although the relation between cigarette smoking and primary hypertension remains uncertain, smoking is a

选的治疗措施应是减轻体重。体重的减轻可使血压下降。肥胖者中的轻型高血压病患者,可用减轻体重的方法纠正高血压。而体重的减轻则是通过减少热量的摄入和增加体力活动得以实现的。对中、重型高血压病患者,减轻体重应同时结合药物治疗。

(二) 限制盐的摄入

限制盐的摄入是治疗高血压的方法之一。现代研究表明,氯化钠的摄入量减少至每日 400 mg 以下时,可以有效地降低血压。对中、重型高血压患者来说,每天钠盐的摄入从 3.5 g 减至 2 g,同时增加钾盐摄入,在几个月之内血压可有轻度的下降,但对轻型高血压病患者采用相同方法尚未证实有明显降压作用,故此方法仅适合短期应用。

(三) 戒烟、少饮酒

吸烟和饮酒与高血压病之间的关系还未能确定,但吸烟是心血管病

chief risk factor of cardiovascular disease. The incidence of coronary heart disease is higher in the smoking hypertensives than in the non-smoking ones by 50% - 60%. Therefore, smokers must be told repeatedly and unambiguously to stop smoking. However, limited intake of alcohol is beneficial, because it may increase the serum level of high-density lipoprotein (HDL) and reduce occurrence of atherosclerosis.

Section Four   Lifestyle Modification

It is recommended that hypertensives should have a regular life adaptable to the change of the natural world. Only in this way can man and nature correspond to each other. Thus healthy-qi is sufficient and diseases would not occur. Otherwise, prolonged disharmony between man and nature may impair genetic material, disturb functional balance, and cause yin deficiency and yang hyperactivity, giving rise to primary hypertension.

的一个主要危险因素。吸烟的高血压病患者,其冠心病发生的危险较不吸烟的高血压病患者增加 50%～60%。因此,对高血压病患者应积极地劝其戒烟。而少量饮酒对高血压病患者是有益的,这可能是通过增加血清高密度脂蛋白胆固醇水平,来减少动脉粥样硬化发生的。

(四)起居有常

起居有常,是指生活要有一定的规律,这种规律还要符合自然界的变化规律。只有这样才能天人相应,正气充盛而不受邪发病。如天人不相应,久之破坏机体遗传物质及多年建立的功能平衡,阴阳失调,阴虚阳亢而发生高血压病。

高血压病的中医特色疗法

Part Three   Experience of Famous Senior TCM Doctors

Chapter One   Zhou Zhongying's Experience

Section One   Understanding of Etiology and Pathogenesis

Zhou Zhongying, a senior doctor of TCM, believes that TCM recognized primary hypertension early in ancient times although there was not a special term known as "hypertension". According to its clinical symptoms, hypertension belongs to diseases of the liver meridian and has close relations with dizziness, headache, syncope or cold limbs, and with liver-yang, liver-fire and liver-wind, and is associated with palpitation and apoplexy to a certain degree. All these are the bases on which the rule of its pathogenesis, syndrome differentiation and treatment can be deduced.

The pathogenesis of primary hypertension, in Zhou's opinion, includes many causative factors and their interactions, and the internal factors are always fundamental.

下篇　名老中医治验

一、周仲瑛治验

（一）病机新识

周仲瑛老中医认为中医学虽无高血压病的名称,但对本病已早有认识,根据其临床症状,主要隶属于肝经病证项下,与眩晕、头痛、厥证、肝阳、肝火、肝风等关系甚为密切,并与心悸、中风有一定联系。这些均是探讨其病理机制及辨证施治规律的依据。

对于高血压病的发病机制,周老认为本病可因情志刺激,五志过极,忧郁恼怒惊恐,思虑过度,持续性精

The factors include emotional stimuli, overacting of five emotional activities, melancholy, anger, terror, anxiety, persistent mental stress; or overeating of peppery, sweet or fat food and overdrinking of alcohol; or indulging in sexual life with exhaustion of vital essence; and excess or deficiency of congenital constitution. After the disease occurs, pathologic changes and syndromes varies with individual constitution, primary causative factors and the changes of disease course, hence, the treatment must be based on syndrome differentiation.

1. The basic pathologic change is the imbalance between yin and yang of the liver, kidney and heart and the hyperactivity of yang and deficiency of yin.

Pathogenic origins can be deduced according to presented symptoms. Although hypertension is mainly manifested as the symptoms of liver meridian, it usually has close relations with the kidney and heart, for internal organs function as a whole. The liver is chiefly involved in the early stage, and the kidney and heart even spleen will be involved later, and the involvement in these organs varies during the course of disease.

Imbalance between yin and yang in zang-fu organs can result in two pathologic changes, i. e. hyperactivity of yang and deficiency of yin. If the disease lasts for a long time, hyperactivity of yang, usually hyperactivity of

神紧张;或饮食不节,嗜食肥甘辛辣,
纵情饮酒;或劳欲过度,精气内伤;或
体质禀赋偏盛、偏虚,如过瘦、过肥等
多种因素及其相互作用所导致,且总
以内因为发病的基础。当其发病之
后,由于素体及原始病因的不同,疾
病先后阶段的演变发展,可以表现多
种病理变化及不同证候,为此,必须
辨证论治。

1. 病理变化主要为肝、肾、心的阴阳失调,阴虚阳亢

审证求因,高血压病虽然表现以
肝经病候为主,但因内脏之间的整体
关系,往往与肾、心密切相关,早期多
以肝为主,以后常见与肾、心同病,且
可涉及到脾,但其间又有主次的
不同。

由于脏腑阴阳平衡失调,表现阳
亢与阴虚两个方面的病变。阳亢主
要为心肝阳亢,但久延可致伤阴,发
展为肝肾阴虚,而肝肾(心)阴虚,阴

heart-yang and liver-yang, may damage yin, leading to deficiency of liver-yin and kidney-yin. The deficient yin in the liver and kidney (and heart) can not restrain the hyperactive yang and further cause hyperactivity of yang in the heart and liver. Yang hyperactivity can cause yin deficiency, and vice versa. Its pathologic change is chiefly "hyperactivity of yang and deficiency of yin" and its clinical manifestation is "deficiency in the lower and excess in the upper". In a small number of cases, yin may damage yang, resulting in deficiency of both yin and yang in the advanced stage.

Secondary excess is the main aspect of the disease at its early stage among the young and middle-aged patients and will gradually develop into yang hyperactivity and yin deficiency, and primary deficiency is the principal aspect in protracted cases. Secondary excess is usually associated with pathogenic wind, fire and phlegm, and primary deficiency is mostly yin deficiency. The normal functional activity of zang-fu organs and yin-yang is the basis of formation and circulation of qi and blood. Imbalance between zang-fu organs or between yin and yang will definitely bring about disorder of qi and blood circulation, which, in turn, aggravates the imbalance between zang-fu organs or yin and yang. In some women cases, pregnancy, multiparity, or menopause may disturb the bal-

不制阳,又可导致心肝阳亢。两者之间互为因果,故其病理中心以"阴虚阳亢"为主,表现"下虚上实"之候。少数患者,后期阴伤及阳,可致阴阳两虚。

　　从其病程经过而言,一般初起及中青年患者以标实居多,逐渐发展为阴虚阳亢,久病不愈又以本虚为主。标实多是风火痰兼挟,本虚多为阴虚。脏腑阴阳的正常功能活动,是生化气血并主宰其运行的基础,脏腑阴阳失调也必然引起气血运行的反常,而气血运行的紊乱又可加重脏腑阴阳的失调。部分妇女患者,因妊娠、多育,或天癸将竭之际,阴阳乖逆,可导致冲任失调。因冲任隶属肝肾,冲为血海,任主一身之阴,而肝藏血,肾藏精,故肝肾阴虚,则冲任失调而为病。

ance between yin and yang, and result in disorder of thoroughfare and conception vessels. Thoroughfare vessel is the sea of blood and conception vessel controls yin of the whole body, and both are attributed to the liver and kidney. Since the liver stores blood and kidney stores essence, deficiency of the liver and kidney may cause the disorder of thoroughfare and conception vessels.

2. The pathologic factors are wind, fire and phlegm, which are concomitant and transformable mutually.

Because of imbalance between zang-fu organs or between yin and yang, yang hyperactivity and yin deficiency not only interact as both cause and effect, but can produce pathologic fire, wind and phlegm, and the three pathologic factors may occur simultaneously and can change into each other. Thus, pathologic changes may take place. For instance, "flaming of fire and stirring up of wind", "fanning fire by pathogenic wind", "stirring up of phlegm by flaming of fire", "stagnated phlegm transforming into fire", and "activating phlegm by stirring up of wind", etc. However, the pathologic changes vary with different cases and different stages of the disease.

Either deficiency of healthy qi or excess of pathogenic factor may predominate in wind, fire or phlegm syndrome. Yang hyperactivity may cause excess of heart-fire

2. 病理因素为风、火、痰,三者可以相互转化、并见

在脏腑阴阳失调的基础上,不但阳亢与阴虚互为因果,且可导致化火、动风、生痰,三者又可相互转化、兼夹,表现"火动风生","风助火势","痰因火动","痰郁化火","风动痰升"等。惟在不同个体及病的不同阶段,又有主次、先后之分。

风、火、痰三者均有偏实、偏虚的不同。凡属阳亢而致心肝火盛,阳化内风,蒸液成痰者属实,久延伤阴,则

and liver-fire and consequently transform into internal wind or broil the body liquid to phlegm, resulting in excess syndrome. If hyperactivity of yang lasts for a long period, it may impair yin, changing the excess syndrome to deficiency syndrome. Yin deficiency may induce the stirring up of endogenous deficient wind and further bring about upward flaming of deficient fire and broil the body liquid into phlegm, resulting in deficiency syndrome. Subsequently, a syndrome of primary deficiency and secondary excess (deficiency syndrome complicated with excess syndrome) may take place.

3. The pathologic outcome is disorder of blood and qi and obstruction of collaterals by blood-stasis when the disease is protracted.

When the disease lasts for a long time or develops rapidly, there may be deficiency of yin in the lower and hyperactivity of yang in the upper. The upward flow of liver-wind, phlegm and fire may disturb qi and blood, causing disorder of qi and blood. Qi runs upwards and blood flows adversely, and even blocks the collaterals and orifices, resulting in fainting or apoplexy. If wind-phlegm invades collaterals, qi and blood are stagnated and collaterals are blocked, resulting in hemiplegia and deviation of eyes and mouth. If heart-meridian is obstructed, obstruction of qi in the chest and precordial pain

由实转虚;因阴虚而致虚风内动,虚火上炎,灼津成痰(或气不化津)者属因虚致实,表现本虚标实(虚中夹实)之证。

3. 久病气血逆乱,可见气升血逆及血瘀络痹的病理转归

如病延日久,或病情急剧发展,虚实向两极分化,阴虚于下,阳亢于上,肝风痰火升腾,冲激气血,气血逆乱,可见气升血逆,甚至阻塞窍络,突发昏厥卒中之变,或风痰入络,气血郁滞,血瘀络痹,而致肢体不遂,偏枯喎僻,或因心脉瘀阻而见胸痹、心痛。

may result.

Section Two   Diagnostic and Therapeutic Characteristics

1. Essentials of treatment based on syndrome differentiation

(1) Determination of pathologic nature: It is necessary to determine whether yang hyperactivity or yin deficiency, secondary excess or primary deficiency is the chief pathologic change, and treatment of suppressing yang or nourishing yin should be employed accordingly. In the case with deficiency of yin affecting yang, a warming and nourishing therapy should be chosen.

(2) Differentiation of pathogenic factors: In the cases with secondary excess as the main syndrome, it is necessary to notice whether wind, fire or phlegm is the chief pathogenic factor, and treatment of subduing wind, purging fire or eliminating phlegm can be used accordingly.

(3) Verification of the pathogenesis and the involved zang-fu organs: In the cases with primary deficiency, it is necessary to determine whether the liver, kidney and heart is chiefly involved, and treatment of nourishing liver, nourishing kidney or nourishing heart should be applied accordingly.

（二）诊疗特色

1. 辨治要点

（1）辨清病理性质：掌握阳亢与阴虚，标实与本虚的主次，予以潜阳、滋阴；阴虚及阳者又当温养。

（2）区别病理因素：标实为主者，分清风、火、痰的主次，予以熄风、清火、化痰。

（3）审察脏腑病机：本虚为主者，鉴别肝、肾、心的重点，予以柔肝、滋肾、养心。

2. Routine treatment

（1） Wind-yang hyperactivity: Dizziness, blurred vision, head distension, headache or dragging pain in temple and vertical regions, flushed face, venule engorgement of head, tinnitus, sounding in the head, restlessness, numbness of limbs, muscular twitching, dry mouth and bitter taste, red tongue with yellow and thin coating, and wiry and rapid pulse.

Treatment: Xifeng Qianyang Fang （decoction）, composed of Gouteng 15 g （decocted later）, Tianma 10 g, Juemingzi 12 g, Yejuhua 10 g, Luobumaye 15 g, Zhenzhumu 30 g （decocted first）, Xuanshen 10 g and Cheqiancao 10 g. Add Chouwutong and Xixiancao for numbness; add Cijili and Chantui for serious dizziness and headache; add Longdancao, Heishanzhizi or Dahuang for flushed face, conjunctival congestion, epistaxis and constipation.

（2） Interior excess of phlegm-fire: Dizziness, heaviness and pain in the head, expectoration of sticky sputum, chest distress, restlessness, fright, obesity, heavy sensation of the body, numbness of the limbs, aphasia, salivation, dry or sticky mouth and bitter taste, yellow and greasy coating, red tip of the tongue, and wiry, smooth and rapid pulse.

Treatment: Qinghuo Huatan Fang （decoction）, composed of Zhulibanxia 10 g, Chendanxing 6 g, Chao-

2. 治疗常规

（1）风阳上亢证：头晕目眩，头胀头痛，或颠顶掣痛，面赤升火，头筋跃起，脑响耳鸣，烦躁，肢麻肉䀼，口干口苦。苔薄黄，舌质红，脉弦数。

【治疗】　熄风潜阳方。钩藤（后下）15 g，天麻10 g，决明子12 g，野菊花10 g，罗布麻叶15 g，珍珠母（先煎）30 g，玄参10 g，车前草10 g。肢麻不利加臭梧桐、豨莶草；头晕痛甚加刺蒺藜、蝉蜕；面红、目赤、鼻衄、便结加龙胆草、黑山栀子或大黄。

（2）痰火内盛证：头晕重痛，咯吐黏痰，胸闷，神烦善惊，形体多肥，身重肢麻，语謇多涎，口干苦或黏。舌苔黄腻，舌尖红，脉弦滑数。

【治疗】　清火化痰方。竹沥半夏10 g，陈胆星6 g，炒黄芩10 g，夏枯

huangqin 10 g, Xiakucao 12 g, Zhibaijiangcan 10 g,
Haizao 10 g, Muli 30 g (decocted first) and Zexie 15 g.
Add Huanglian and Fushen for vexation and dreaminess;
and Yujin and Tianzhuhuang for mental derangement;
add Gualou and Fenghuaxiao for chest distress, abundant
expectoration and constipation.

(3) Qi and blood disorder: Head distension, headache or stabbing pain of head, lusterless complexion, feverish face, oppressed sensation or stinging pain in the
chest, occasional palpitation, wandering pain of limbs,
irregular menstruation, dry mouth, darkish tongue with
thin coating or with petechiae and ecchymosis, and
thready, unsmooth or irregular pulse.

Treatment: Tiaoqi Hexue Fang (decoction), composed of Danshen 12 g, Chuanxiong 10 g, Daji 15 g,
Xiaoji 15 g, Huainiuxi 10 g, Shenghuaimi 10 g, Guangdilong 10 g and Daizheshi 25 g. Add Cijili for dizziness;
add Gegen for neck rigidity; add Gualoupi and
Pianjianghuang for oppressed feeling and pain in the
chest; add Jixueteng and Honghua for numbness of limbs;
add Chaihu and Xuchangqing for fullness and distension
in the chest and hypochondrium or wandering pain of
limbs; add Chongweizi for irregular menstruation.

(4) Liver-yin and kidney-yin deficiency: Dizziness,
headache, dry eyes and blurred vision, tinnitus, flushed

草12 g,炙白僵蚕10 g,海藻10 g,牡蛎
(先煎)30 g,泽泻15 g。心烦梦多加黄
连、茯神;神情异常加郁金、天竺黄;
胸闷、痰多、便秘加瓜蒌、风化硝。

(3)气血失调证：头痛头胀,或
痛处如针刺,面色黯红,时有烘热,胸
部有紧压感,或胸痛如刺,间有心悸,
肢体窜痛或顽麻,妇女月经不调,口
干。苔薄,舌质偏黯,或有紫点、瘀
斑,脉或细,或涩,或结代。

【治疗】　调气和血方。丹参
12 g,川芎10 g,大蓟、小蓟各15 g,怀
牛膝10 g,生槐米10 g,广地龙10 g,代
赭石25 g。头昏加刺蒺藜;颈项强急加
葛根;胸闷胸痛加瓜蒌皮、片姜黄;肢
麻不利加鸡血藤、红花;胸胁满胀或
窜痛加柴胡、徐长卿;妇女月经不调
加茺蔚子。

(4)肝肾阴虚证：头昏晕痛,目
涩视糊,耳鸣,遇劳则面赤升火,肢

高血压病的中医特色疗法

face with hot sensation under physical exertion, numbness of limbs, sore lumbus and weak legs, dry mouth, red tongue with little coating, and thready and wiry or thready and rapid pulse.

Treatment: Zirou Ganshen Fang (decoction), composed of Dashengdihuang 15 g, Gouqizi 10 g, Zhinüzhenzi 10 g, Zhiheshouwu 12 g, Sangjisheng 12 g, Shengshijueming 30 g (decocted first), Juhua 10 g and Cijili 10 g. Add Muli and Biejia for dizziness and flushed face; add Zhimu and Huangbai for restlessness and fever; add Baishaoyao for numbness of limbs; add Suanzaoren and Ejiao for insomnia and dreaminess.

(5) **Yin deficiency affecting yang**: Dizziness, blurred vision, dim eyesight, pale and lustreless complexion, occasional fever, spiritlessness, shortness of breath, cold extremities and body, sore lumbus, weak limbs, nocturnal urination, enlarged and reddish or pale tongue, and sunken and thready pulse.

Treatment: Wenyang Ganshen Fang (decoction), composed of Yinyanghuo 10 g, Roucongrong 10 g, Danggui 10 g, Dashudihuang 12 g, Gouqizi 10 g, Duzhong 12 g, Lingcishi (decocted first) 20 g and Huangbai 5 g. Add Shayuanzi for dizziness and dim eyesight; add Shenghuangqi and Wuweizi for palpitation and shortness of breath; add Dang-shen and Huaishanyao for lassitude and

麻,腰酸腿软,口干。舌红少苔,脉细弦或细数。

【治疗】　滋柔肝肾方。大生地黄15 g,枸杞子10 g,炙女贞子10 g,制何首乌12 g,桑寄生12 g,生石决明(先煎)30 g,菊花10 g,刺蒺藜10 g。头眩、面色潮红加牡蛎、鳖甲;烦热加知母、黄柏;肢麻加白芍药;失眠多梦加酸枣仁、阿胶。

(5) 阴虚及阳证:头昏,目花,视糊,面白少华,间有烘热,神疲气短,腰酸腿软,肢清足冷,夜尿频数。舌淡红或淡白,质胖,脉沉细。

【治疗】　温养肝肾方。淫羊藿10 g,肉苁蓉10 g,当归10 g,大熟地黄12 g,枸杞子10 g,杜仲12 g,灵磁石(先煎)20 g,黄柏5 g。头昏目花加沙苑子;心悸气短加生黄芪、五味子;倦怠、大便不实加党参、怀山药;怯寒、足肿加制附子、白术。

loose stool; add Zhifuzi and Baizhu for aversion to cold
and edema of leg.

3. Six methods of syndrome differentiation and treatments

(1) Liver-wind can move upwards and sideways and
therefore deficiency-type and excess-type should be dis-
tinguished.

Liver-wind results from hyperactivity of liver-yang
and induces two pathologic changes. Firstly, it attacks
vertex, manifested as dragging pain in the head, seasick-
ness-like dizziness, tinnitus, dim eyesight and even sudden falling down in a faint. It should be treated by suppressing hyperactive yang and wind with drugs such as
Tianma, Gouteng, Cijili, Juhua, Luobumaye, Shijueming, Longchi, Muli, Zhenzhumu, and Lingyangjiao, etc.
Secondly, it moves sideways and invades collaterals,
manifested as numbness of limbs, convulsion, slight muscular twitching, neck rigidity, aphasia, and even hemiplegia, and should be treated by expelling wind and activating collaterals with drugs such as Xixiancao, Dilong,
Quanxiewei, Baijiangcan, Chouwutong, etc.

As to wind-yang hyperactivity, it results from failure
of the kidney and the blood to nourish the liver. On one
hand, it may be manifested as dizziness, numbness of
limbs, which are induced by internal disturbance of

3. 证治六辨

(1) 肝风有上冒和旁走之分、虚实之辨：肝风是由于肝阳亢盛所致，在病理反映上有两类情况：一是肝风上冒巅顶，表现为头部掣痛、眩晕，如坐舟车，耳鸣目花，甚则一时性厥仆，治当熄风潜阳，用天麻、钩藤、刺蒺藜、菊花、罗布麻叶、石决明、龙齿、牡蛎、珍珠母、羚羊角之类。另一是肝风旁走入络，表现为肢体麻木、抽搐、肌肉𬌗动、项强、语謇，甚则瘫痪不遂，治当祛风和络，用豨莶草、地龙、全蝎尾、白僵蚕、臭梧桐等。

至于风阳亢盛，由于水不涵木、血不养肝而致者，虽有眩晕、肢麻等虚风内动之候，但必具肝肾阴虚之征，如头昏目涩、视物模糊、虚烦、颧

deficiency-fire. On the other hand, it is inevitably manifested as dizziness, blurred vision, vexation, flushed
cheeks, lumbago, weakness of limbs, red tongue,
thready and wiry pulse, which are induced by deficiency
of liver-yin and kidney-yin. It should be treated by
replenishing kidney-yin and nourishing the liver, so as to
suppress hyperactivity of endogenous wind. This is somewhat different from the method of suppressing hyperactive wind and yang, which is simply used for the excess
syndrome due to hyperactivity of yang and stirring-up of
endogenous wind. Clinically, for cases with failure of
kidney to nourish the liver, Shengdihuang, Xuanshen,
Ejiao, Nüzhenzi, Sangshenzi, Muli, Guiban, Zhibiejia, etc.
should be used to nourish the kidney and liver or nourish yin
and suppress yang. For the case with yin-blood deficiency and
blood failing to nourish the liver, Danggui, Dihuang,
Baishaoyao, Gouqizi, Heshouwu, Heizhima, etc. should be
applied to nourish blood, sooth the liver, suppress wind and
activate collaterals. These two categories of drugs are often
combined for use, but the proportion between them should be
carefully determined when a prescription is made. Drugs for
suppressing and eliminating wind should be added properly at
the same time.

(2) Phlegm syndrome can be classified into phlegm-
fire, wind-phlegm or turbid-phlegm type.

红、腰膝酸软、舌质红、脉细弦等。在治疗上应以滋水涵木为主,以达到平息内风的目的,与阳亢风动、单纯用熄风潜阳法的实证有所不同。具体言之,水不涵木者,当滋肾养肝,育阴潜阳,用生地黄、玄参、阿胶、女贞子、桑椹子、牡蛎、龟版、炙鳖甲等品。若阴血不足,血不养肝者,又当养血柔肝以熄风和络,用当归、地黄、白芍药、枸杞子、何首乌、黑芝麻等品。以上两类药物虽多交叉合用,但组方时应把握其主次比例,同时佐以熄风或祛风之品。

（2）痰证当辨痰火、风痰、痰浊之异：痰盛者,一般多兼火象,上犯头目

Overabundance of phlegm is often associated with fire. That attacking the head and eyes is manifested as dizziness and headache; and that disturbing the mind as mental derangement, restlessness, fright, dementia, soliloquy and emotional upset. It should be treated by clearing fire and dissipating phlegm. Huanglian Wendan Tang (decoction), Mengshi Guntan Wan (pill) or Xuegeng Tang (decoction) are used by adding Dannanxing, Tianzhuhuang, Zhuli, Haizao and Fenghuaxiao, etc. In the case of phlegm combined with wind, symptoms of wind stirring and phlegm rising (dizziness) and of wind-phlegm attacking collaterals (numbness of limbs, heavy sensation of the body, stiffness of the tongue, and aphasia), Banxia Tianma Baizhu Tang (decoction) with additions of Baijiangcan, Nanxing and Baifuzi should be applied, or Zhimi Fuling Wan (pill) is indicated at the same time. When turbid phlegm is predominant without signs of fire, the following symtoms may be seen, such as obesity, chest distress, shortness of breath, excessive thick and white sputum with difficult expectoration, nausea, excessive salivation, drowsiness, sticky feeling in the mouth, stiffness of the tongue, white and greasy coating, deep and smooth pulse. It should be treated by drying dampness, resolving phlegm, eliminating turbid phlegm and removing obstruction, and recipes such as Erchen

则头晕痛、目眩,内犯心神则神情异
常、心烦易惊、呆钝、独语、喜哭无常,
治当清火化痰,用黄连温胆汤、礞石
滚痰丸、雪羹汤合胆南星、天竺黄、竹
沥、海藻、风化硝之类;若痰与风合,
可表现风动痰升而见眩晕,又因风痰
入络而致肢体麻木、重着不遂、舌强
语謇,治应祛风化痰,取半夏天麻白
术汤意配白僵蚕、南星、白附子之类,
或另吞指迷茯苓丸。若表现为痰浊
之候,而无明显火象者,其症形体多
肥,面色黄,头昏重,胸闷气短,痰多
黏白,咯吐不利,嗜睡,泛恶,口黏多
涎,舌强不和,苔白腻,脉沉滑。治当
燥湿化痰、泄浊开痹,可用二陈汤、瓜
蒌薤白半夏汤等。气逆加旋覆花、紫
苏子;嗜卧加南星、石菖蒲、远志、矾
郁金。这类证候,有的可进一步化
火,但在本质上,每与脾气虚弱有关,
若久延脾虚之症趋向明显者,当转予
甘温补脾以治本。

Tang (decoction), Gualou Xiebai Banxia Tang (decoction) should be chosen. Xuanfuhua and Zisuzi should be added for the case with upward flow of lung-qi; and Nanxing, Shichangpu, Yuanzhi and Fanyujin for drowsiness. Although this kind of syndrome can transform into fire type, essentially, it has a close relationship with deficiency of spleen-qi. In addition, if the sign of deficiency of spleen-qi becomes apparent, strengthening the spleen with sweet-warm drugs may serve as the primary treatment.

(3) Excessive fire syndrome should be treated by purging liver-fire or purging heart-fire and kidney-fire accordingly.

Excess of fire results mainly from hyperfunction of the liver and should be treated by clearing away liver-heat and purging fire with bitter-cold drugs. Heat-clearing method is effective for mild cases and Mudanpi, Shanzhizi, Huangqin, Xiakucao, Huaihua, Cheqianzi, Zexie, etc. can be used; fire-purging method must be employed for serious cases, and Longdancao, Dahuang, Juemingzi, etc. are needed for the treatment. If fire results from stagnation of liver-qi, it should be treated by dispersing liver-qi with Chaihu, Cijili and Chuanlianzi. On the other hand, attention should be paid to the pathologic relation of the liver with the heart and kidney. In the case that excess of child-organ is caused by the disorder of the mother-organ, manifested as restlessness, irritability, in-

（3）火盛者有清肝泻火与兼泄心肾之别：火盛主要由于肝旺，故治当苦寒泄降，清肝泻火。病势轻者清之即平，如牡丹皮、山栀子、黄芩、夏枯草、槐花、车前子、泽泻之类；重者非泻不降，可用龙胆草、大黄、决明子等品。火起于郁者，还当注意佐以疏泄，酌配柴胡、刺蒺藜、川楝子。另一方面，还当注意肝与心、肾的病理关系。若心烦易怒，寐差多梦，母令子实者，当本着"实则泻其子"的治法，配合泻心的黄连、莲子心。同时因相火生于肾而寄于肝，如下焦相火偏盛，而致肝火上炎者，又当兼泻相火，配合知母、黄柏之类。

somnia and dreaminess, the principle of "purging the child-organ in the case of excess" should be observed and drugs for purging heart-fire such as Huanglian, and Lianzixin should be used. If ministerial fire in lower-energizer is excessive, it would cause flaming up of liver-fire, for ministerial fire originates from the kidney and exists in the liver. In this case, the method of purging ministerial fire may be used complementarily, and drugs such as Zhimu and Huangbo should be added.

(4) Purging fire or nourishing yin should be applied according to individual cases.

In the case of hyperactivity of liver-yang, the routine treatment is to use bitter-cold drugs to purge fire. But prolonged existence of liver-fire inevitably consumes liver-yin and kidney-yin, then liver-fire is the temporary secondary excess, yin deficiency is the primary deficiency. Therefore, bitter-cold drugs should be used with yin-nourishing drugs, otherwise, they may induce pathogenic dryness and impair yin. In some protracted cases with obvious secondary excess, if purging method is not effective, it is probably "deficiency accompanied by excess", for the primary deficiency is covered up by the secondary excess. For the case with obvious yin deficiency, it should be treated mainly by nourishing liver-yin and kidney-yin, based on the principle of "tonifying the

（4）注意辨别泻火与滋阴的应用：肝阳偏亢者,苦寒直折虽为正治,但肝火燔灼日久,终必耗伤肝肾之阴,肝火仅是暂时性的标实,阴虚才是根本性的原因,故苦寒泻火之法,可暂而不可久,宜与甘寒滋阴药配合,而不宜单用。若久用、单用苦寒药而不加佐治,则苦从燥化,反致伤阴;若病程已久,标实症状虽然比较突出,但泻之不应者,可能为虚中夹实,因标实掩盖了本虚的一面。如表现明显阴伤之证,当以滋养肝肾为主,从"虚则补母"考虑,益其肾阴,用知柏地黄丸、大补阴丸之类,杞菊地黄丸、复方首乌丸亦可酌情选用。心阴虚者合补心丹,药如天门冬、麦门

mother-organ in the case of deficiency ", and recipes such as Zhibo Dihuang Wan (pill) and Dabuyin Wan (pill) as well as Qiju Dihuang Wan (pill) and Fufang Shouwu Wan (pill) should be used accordingly. For heart-yin deficiency, Buxin Dan (pill), composed of Tianmendong, Maimendong, Yuzhu, Huangjing, Baiziren, and Suanzaoren, etc. should be applied. In the cases with obvious excessive fire, though bitter-cold drugs are effective in purging fire, yin-nourishing drugs should also be used to avoid relapse.

(5) It is important to decide the proper treatment for qi-blood disorder induced by yin-yang disharmony.

Zang-fu and yin-yang disharmony inevitably causes qi-blood disorder. Since qi is the commander of blood, qi stagnation inevitably causes blood obstruction. On the other hand, blood circulation disorder will bring about failure of qi to ascend and descend. And smooth flow of qi ensures smooth circulation of blood, and vice versa. Hence, it is advisable to combine the method of regulating qi with that of regulating blood. Since hypertensive patients are usually characterized by yang hyperactivity with yin deficiency, for regulating qi, aromatic-acrid drugs should be avoided, while for regulating blood, cool-demulcent drugs are suggested and blood-stasis-removing drugs should be avoided. The liver controls dispersion and stores blood, and is closely related to qi and blood. So it

冬、玉竹、黄精、柏子仁、酸枣仁等。即使在实火明显的情况下,经用苦寒泻火药得效后,亦当滋养肝肾心阴,以谋巩固,否则仅能取效一时,而易于反复。

（5）辨阴阳失调导致气血紊乱之治：脏腑阴阳失调,必然导致气血失调。因为气为血之帅,气有一息之不运,则血有一息之不行,血行紊乱,又碍气机之升降,故调气与和血两相配伍,气调则血和,血和气亦顺。由于高血压病患者多为阴虚阳亢之体,故调气应避免香燥辛散,和血多用凉润和平,忌破血。肝主疏泄,又主藏血,与气血关系最密,且为本病的主病之脏,故调气以平降、疏利肝气为要,和血亦多选入肝之品。由于气血失调是多种因素所导致的病理变化,且每与风阳痰火相因为患,故调气和血常与熄风、潜阳、清火、化痰诸法配合使用。但须按其主次选方用药。病缘

is the main involved organ in primary hypertension. The treatment is hence chiefly to regulate qi and calm the liver and drugs attributable to liver-meridian are used for regulating blood. Since qi and blood disorder results from various pathogenic factors and is usually associated with wind-yang and phlegm-fire, regulating qi and blood is often applied with calming wind, suppressing yang, dispersing fire and resolving phlegm. Clinically, these methods should be used in accordance with individual cases. Furthermore, in the case with healthy-qi deficiency, the method of regulating qi and blood should be combined with that of invigorating qi and nourishing blood.

For the case with liver-qi stagnation, which is manifested as distending pain and oppressed sensation in the chest and hypochondrium, wandering pain of the body, it should be treated by regulating qi and alleviating depression. Based on the principle of Danzhi Xiaoyao San (powder), use Chaihu, Cijili, Yujin, Lü'emei plus Mudanpi, Shanzhizi, Huangqin, etc. to disperse stagnant qi and fire in the liver meridian. This therapy is very effective for those accompanied by mental stress. For the case with stirring-up of qi and blood, manifested as heaviness of the head, weak legs, flushed face, and venule engorgement in temple, it should be treated by inducing qi and blood downward with the drugs as Huainiuxi, Chong-

正虚者,又当与养血、益气等补益法配合。

如肝气郁结,胸胁苦闷痹痛,气不得展,周身窜痛者,须理气解郁,仿丹栀逍遥散,用柴胡、刺蒺藜、郁金、绿萼梅,配合牡丹皮、山栀子、黄芩等升散肝经郁结的气火。此法施之于有精神紧张症状者其合拍。气血上逆,头重腿软,面赤,颞部筋脉跃起者,当顺降气血,诱导下行,用怀牛膝、茺蔚子、大蓟、小蓟、灵磁石、代赭石等药。血瘀络痹,四肢麻木者,当活血和络,用鸡血藤、当归须、赤芍药、红花、桑寄生之类。若心血瘀阻,胸膺闷痛,唇黯舌紫者当以化瘀通

weizi, Daji, Xiaoji, Lingcishi and Daizheshi. For the case with meridian obstruction due to blood-stasis, characterized by numbness of limbs, it should be treated by promoting blood circulation to remove meridian obstruction, use Jixueteng, Dangguixu, Chishaoyao, Honghua and Sangjisheng. For the case with heart-blood stagnation manifested as stuffy pain in the chest, dull purple lips, and purple tongue, it should be treated by resolving blood-stasis to remove meridian obstruction, use Taoren, Honghua, Danshen, Chuanxiong, Jianghuang, Ruxiang, Shixiaosan (i.e. Puhuang and Wulingzhi), Shanzha. This method is suitable for those associated with hypertensive heart disease or coronary sclerosis.

(6) Warming kidney and reinforcing spleen should be applied based on the differentiation between spleen-deficiency and kidney-deficiency.

Warming yang and reinforcing qi is usually used for primary hypertension at advanced stage. In protracted cases yin impairment involves yang, leading to yang-deficiency. At this stage, the case, though with a high blood pressure, is manifested as symptoms of yang insufficiency. Hence, bitter-cool or yin-nourishing drugs would not be effective, and if used they may impair or obstruct yang-qi. Therefore, the treatment must be based on the general condition of the case other than on blood pressure

脉,用桃仁、红花、丹参、川芎、姜黄、乳香、失笑散、山楂等品,如检查有高血压心脏病或冠状动脉硬化者可采用之。

(6)辨温补脾肾变法之应用:温阳补气法多为高血压病后期,病程日久,阴伤及阳,导致阳虚变证的变治方法。此时血压虽高,但其全身症状,主要表现为阳气不足,因此,已非苦寒或单纯滋阴方法所能取效,误用反致伤害和抑遏阳气,必须从整体分析,防止单从血压考虑。温补法的具体运用,则当区别脾虚和肾虚的不同,分别处理。脾气虚者,多见于肥胖之人,形盛气衰,"土不栽木"而致风木自动,一方面积湿生痰停饮,而

alone. In addition, spleen-deficiency or kidney-deficiency should be differentiated, when warming method is applied. Spleen-qi deficiency is mostly seen in obese patient whose physique is strong but qi is insufficient. "Earth failing to nourish wood" would induce wind-wood moving, which on one hand, causes dampness-accumulation and phlegm-retention, manifested as the secondary excess as "qi deficiency and phlegm excess"; and on the other hand, causes middle-energizer qi deficiency and spleen-yang insufficiency, manifested as shortness of breath, weakness, dizziness, abundant expectoration, nausea, indigestion, loose stool, pale tongue with white and greasy coating, and weak pulse, especially seen in protracted cases. When secondary excess is significant, phlegm-resolving method should be employed, but when primary deficiency is predominant, spleen-tonifying method should be used, togeter with sweet-warm drugs such as Dangshen, Huangqi, Fuling, and Baizhu, so as to strengthen spleen-qi and eliminate phlegm. This method based on the principle of Liujunzi Tang (decoction) aims at replenishing the spleen to nourish the liver. As to the case with obvious fluid-retention, manifested as aversion to cold, palpitation, vomiting and edema, it should be treated together with Linggui Zhugan Tang (decoction) to warm yang and remove fluid-retention. This syndrome may be seen in the case of hypertensive heart disease associated with heart failure.

见标实之候，表现为"气虚痰盛"；另一方面又见中气不足、脾阳衰弱的虚象，表现气短、倦怠、头眩、痰多、泛恶、食后不运、大便不实、舌淡、苔白腻、脉软等症，其病程久延之后，则尤为明显。当标实为主时，固当化痰，但如虚象为主时，就必须用甘温补脾之法，予党参、黄芪、茯苓、白术之类，补气以杜痰源，兼以化痰治标，仿六君子汤意培土栽木；若饮象明显，畏寒、心悸、呕吐痰涎、浮肿者，应合苓桂术甘汤以温阳化饮。这类证候可见于高血压心脏病伴有心力衰竭之患者。

As the disease progresses, liver-yin and kidney-yin deficiency ultimately results in kidney-yang deficiency, thus, not only water in yin but fire in yin may be deficient, leading to kidney fire failing to return to its residence and deficient yang floating in the upper. This is manifested as dizziness, dim eyesight, nocturnal urination, unsteady steps, enlarged and delicate tongue, sunken and thready pulse and as well, impotence in man and irregular menstruation in woman. It should be treated by warming and nourishing kidney-qi, and suppressing deficient yang. Furthermore, yang originates from yin, when yin impairs yang, it is advisable to invigorate both yang and yin. In this case, Jingui Shenqi Wan (pill) should be used as the basic recipe. In this prescription, Fuzi and Guizhi, the main drugs, though acrid in taste and warm in nature, exert a potent effect of warming yang and promoting blood circulation. Moreover, because of its cordial effect, Fuzi is particularly effective for the case at the later stage of hypertension with deficiency of heart- and kidney-yang. Women with irregular menstruation, resulting from disharmony between thoroughfare and conception vessels, should be treated with Erxian Tang (decoction) (Xianmao, Xianlingpi, Danggui, Bajitian, Huangbai, and Zhimu) along with Duzhong, Roucongrong, Sangjisheng, Chongweizi, etc. This decoction, if

肾阳虚属肝肾阴虚后期进一步的发展,此时不但阴中之水虚,同时阴中之火亦虚,以致火不归宅,虚阳浮越于上,上则头目昏眩,下则足冷,夜尿频数,步履飘浮,舌质胖嫩,脉象沉细,男子阳痿,女子月经不调,治当温养肾气,潜纳虚阳。同时由于阴阳互根,今阴伤及阳,故当兼予补阴以配阳,可以金匮肾气丸为基础方。阴阳并补,方中附桂虽属辛温,但可藉其温阳之力以助血脉之循行,附子功能强心,故对高血压病后期心肾阳衰者,尤有较好的作用。若妇女因肝肾不足而冲任不调,月经失常者,可用二仙汤(仙茅、仙灵脾、当归、巴戟天、黄柏、知母)及杜仲、肉苁蓉、桑寄生、茺蔚子之类。二仙汤对妇女更年期高血压病见肾阳不振之证者,若用之得当,可有极为明显的疗效。临床试用于男性高血压病证见肾阳虚者,部分病例血压亦可获得大幅度的下降。此即叶桂之温养肝肾法,但须注意去刚用柔。此外,在用大队补阳滋阴剂时,当少佐知母、黄柏等苦寒泄降之品,以制温药刚燥之性,避免助阳太

used in a right way, is very effective for climacteric hypertensive women with kidney-yang deficiency. It was experimentally used in clinic for male hypertensive patients with kidney-yang deficiency, and blood pressure was markedly lowered in some cases. Furthermore, while a number of drugs for warming yang and nourishing yin are used, some bitter-cold drugs, such as Zhimu or Huangbo which has a dispersing or purging property, should be added to restrict their dry and hot nature, so as to avoid damage to yin-essence. In fact, the therapeutic principle of "contrary treatment" is used here, which is beneficial to induce deficient yang down.

4. Clinical experience

(1) Pay attention to pathological changes and individual differences.

On the basis of syndrome differentiation, hypertension can be classified into wind-yang hyperactivity, interior excess of phlegm-fire, qi and blood disorder, liver- and kidney-yin deficiency and yin deficiency affecting yang. This classification is in accord with most cases and beneficial to standardization of treatment. Clinically, the differentiation should be based on the main symptoms rather than on every aspect. When different syndromes are mingled with each other, their relatively stabilizing and inter-transforming relationship should be considered.

过,反致伤阴。同时,还寓有"从治"之意,有利于诱导虚阳的潜降。

4. 临证体会

(1)分证治疗必须注意病情的动态变化与个体差异:高血压病从风阳上亢、痰火内盛、气血失调、肝肾阴虚、阴虚及阳五类证候辨治,可以适用于大多数病例,有助于诊治的规范化。但临证应当综合判断,辨证不必诸症悉具,只要从中找出主症特点,即可作为定证依据,同时必须重视证候的交叉错杂,兼顾并治,注意证型的相对稳定和演变转化的两重性,而药随证转是非常必要的。而在诊治常规的基础上,针对个体差异,相应

On the basis of the routine treatment, it is necessary to modify the prescription according to individual cases, so as to ensure a more satisfactory curative result.

(2) Regulate yin and yang to reduce blood pressure, relieve symptoms and retard the progress of the disease.

Blood pressure elevation is caused by yin and yang disharmony. Clinically, various therapeutic methods or prescriptions used to regulate yin and yang are effective for decreasing blood pressure, maintaining it in an acceptable range. In most patients, alleviation of symptoms usually follows with reduction of blood pressure. But in some cases, particularly in later stage, blood pressure may still remain high even after a long period of treatment. However, the treatment can obviously improve the condition of disease, which means that disharmony of yin and yang is greatly improved and hence the progress of disease is retarded.

(3) Treat the coexistence of secondary excess and primary deficiency.

Primary deficiency and secondary excess are the two pathologic aspects of primary hypertension. The former can bring about the latter and vice versa. Yin deficiency and yang hyperactivity are the two contradictory aspects which oppose and affect each other. Therefore, in treatment, attention should be paid to both aspects, and yang-

变通组方配药,将更有利于疗效的提高。

(2)调整阴阳,可以降低血压,改善临床症状,延缓病情进展:血压升高是机体阴阳的动态平衡失调所致。临床采用各种治法方药,调节阴阳归之于平,常可有效地降低血压,而且对巩固降压疗效起积极作用。临床所见,改善症状与降低血压的疗效并不完全一致,多数病例症状减轻而血压亦降。部分患者,特别是后期病例,经长期治疗虽自觉症状显减或基本消失,但血压仍处于高于正常的状态,但症状改善却标志着阴阳平衡失调有所纠正,这对延缓或阻止病情的发展,是有一定作用的。

(3)标实与本虚每多错杂,治当酌情兼顾:本病有虚有实,标实可导致本虚,本虚又可产生标实,阴虚和阳亢是矛盾对立、互为影响的两个方面,因此,在治疗时原则上应当标本兼顾。予以潜阳、滋阴,针对具体情况区别主次施治。一般病程不长,年壮体实,标症为急者,多以治标为主;

suppressing or yin-nourishing method should be used properly according to individual cases. Generally, for the cases with a short course and of strong constitution and in a condition that secondary excess is predominant, the principle is to treat secondary excess. But for protracted cases in the elderly with obvious deficiency, the principle is to treat the primary deficiency. At the same time, the treatment should be adjusted according to the pathological changes or changes between the deficiency and the excess.

Three pathogenic factors, wind, fire and phlegm, which result in secondary excess, usually mix with and change into each other, so therapeutic methods of suppressing wind, clearing fire and dissipating phlegm are often used together. As soon as secondary syndromes have been relieved or excessive syndrome changes into deficient one because of protraction of the disease, proper treatment should be applied for primary deficiency in order to protect healthy-qi. Although primary deficiency is classified into deficiency of the liver, kidney and heart, they can affect each other and even take place in the meantime. Deficiency of liver-yin and blood may result in hyperactivity of yang and fire, and further damage the heart and kidney, causing simultaneous dysfunction of the liver and kidney, of the heart and liver, or of the heart

久病下虚明显,年龄较大者,则以治本为主。同时当随着先后阶段病理的演变、虚实的转化相应处理。

引起标实的风、火、痰三者既多错综并见,又易互为影响演变,因此,熄风、清火、化痰常需综合使用。一旦标证缓解,或久延由实转虚,就应重点转向治本,不宜攻伐太过。至于本虚,虽有肝、肾、心等区别,但亦互有影响,兼夹并病。由于肝的阴血不足,阳亢火旺,而上炎于心,下病及肾,常表现肝肾、心肝、心肾同病。因此,柔肝、滋肾、养心,亦多兼顾并施。此外,肝脾、肝肺同病,表现土不栽木,脾湿生痰,风木内动;或肝火犯肺,金不制木,风火上炎者,又当熄风化痰,培土栽木,或清金制木。

and kidney. Therefore, therapeutic methods of soothing the liver, nourishing the kidney and reinforcing the heart are often used together. In addition, pathologic changes of the liver and spleen or of the liver and lung may happen simultaneously, characterized by the earth failing to nourish wood, spleen dampness producing phlegm, and stirring-up of wind-wood, or by liver-fire attacking lung, metal failing to restrict wood, and flaming up of wind-fire. For these cases, the method of suppressing wind and resolving phlegm, replenishing earth to nourish wood, or clearing the lung to restrain the liver should be employed accordingly.

Section Three   Typical Cases

He, male, aged 38, a cadre.

First visit: Dec. 18, 1993.

He had suffered from dizziness for 5 months, and was diagnosed as hypertension and hyperlipemia. Many western and Chinese medicines were administered but were not effective. He experienced dizziness, and even headache sometimes, chest distress, pain in the shoulder and back, and numbness of left upper limb. His tongue was red with little coating, pulse thready and rapid. He is fat, body weight 72 kg, and height 1.67 m. Physical examination revealed that TG 3.8 mmol/L; TC, 7.8 mmol/L;

（三）验案举隅

何某某,男,38 岁,干部。1993年 12 月 18 日初诊。

眩晕 5 月,查为高血压、高脂血症,经多种中西医药物治疗不效。现眩晕,头昏时痛,心胸部位常有闷塞不舒,肩背隐痛,左上肢麻木,舌质红,苔少,脉细数。体胖,体重72 kg,身高1.67 m,TG(甘油三酯)3.8 mmol/L,TC(总胆固醇)7.8 mmol/L,BP(血压)22.7/13.3 kPa,ECG(心电图)示偶发早搏。

高血压病的中医特色疗法

BP, 22.7/13.3 kPa. ECG showed occasional premature beat.

Syndrome differentiation: Deficiency of the liver and kidney, stagnation of phlegm and blood stasis, stirring-up of wind-yang.

Therapeutic principle: Nourish the kidney and liver, resolve phlegm, promote blood circulation, calm the liver and suppress wind.

Prescription: Modified Gouteng Yin (decoction) and Jiangzhi Fang Ⅱ (decoction) (the latter was worked out by Zhou himself, composed of Zhiheshouwu, Gouqizi, Sangjisheng, Zexie and Juemingzi, etc.), composed of Tianma 10 g, Gouteng (decocted later) 15 g, Shayuanzi 10 g, Cijili 10 g, Zhihuangjing 10 g, Zhiheshouwu 10 g, Shengshanzharou 12 g, Zexie 15 g, Juemingzi 12 g, Danshen 12 g, Muli 25 g (decocted first), Sangjisheng 15 g and Zhibaijiangcan 10 g.

Second visit: Treated for one month by nourishing the kidney and liver, resolving phlegm and removing blood-stasis, all the symptoms were alleviated except dizziness and numbness of upper limbs. ECG showed sinus bradycardia (56 beats per minute). Reexamination revealed the levels of blood-lipid and blood pressure were lower than before; TG, 2.8 mmol/L; TC, 6.9 mmol/L; BP, 20.67/12.3 kPa. The previous prescription was mo-

【辨证】 肝肾不足，痰瘀阻滞，风阳上扰。

【治法】 滋肾养肝，化痰活血，平肝熄风。

【处方】 钩藤饮合降脂Ⅱ号方（周老自拟方：制何首乌、枸杞子、桑寄生、泽泻、决明子等）加减，天麻10 g，钩藤（后下）15 g，沙苑子10 g，刺蒺藜10 g，制黄精10 g，制何首乌10 g，生山楂肉12 g，泽泻15 g，决明子12 g，丹参12 g，牡蛎（先煎）25 g，桑寄生15 g，炙白僵蚕10 g。

【复诊】 滋肾养肝合化痰祛瘀，药服一月，诸症皆有改善，但眩晕未能全部消失，上肢麻减未已，复查心电图示窦性心动过缓（56 次/分），血脂、血压均呈下降趋势。复查 TG 2.8 mmol/L，TC 6.9 mmol/L，BP 20.67/12.3 kPa，原方去沙苑子刺蒺藜，决明子，加罗布麻叶15 g，菊花

dified by removing Shayuanzi, Cijili, Juemingzi and adding Luobumaye 15 g, Juhua 10 g and Xiakucao 10 g.

Third visit: The condition was stabilized, and dizziness was not obvious. Body weight was reduced by about 3 kg. Fullness of abdomen was relieved. Blood pressure fluctuated within the high range of normal limit; TG, 2.4 mmol/L; TC, 4.2 mmol/L; BP, 18.7/12.0 kPa; ECG, normal. The previous modified prescription was applied for another 3 months.

Fourth visit: All symptoms disappeared except occasional dizziness, blood pressure and blood-lipid remained normal, and body weight reduced by 4.5 kg. The same therapeutic principle was still adopted, and the prescription was composed of Tianma 10 g, Juhua 10 g, Zhiheshouwu 12 g, Gouqizi 10 g, Shengshanzharou 15 g, Juemingzi 10 g, Zexie 15 g, Zhibaijiangcan 10 g, Heye 15 g, Sangjisheng 12 g and Shengmuli 30 g (decocted first).

Follow-up: No recurrence was observed in the following 3 months. The body weight reduced continuously and the patient was satisfied with the curative result. In the prescription for this case, Huangjing, Heshouwu and Sangjisheng were used for nourishing the liver and kidney; Shengshanzha and Danshen for promoting blood circulation and removing blood-stasis; Baijiangcan,

10 g,夏枯草10 g,继进。

三诊:病情稳定,眩晕不著,体重下降约 3 kg,原有脘腹胀塞感转为宽松,血压波动于正常高界范围,复查EGG 正常,血脂 TG 2.4 mmol/L,TC 4.2 mmol/L,BP 18.7/12.0 kPa,续服上药 3 个月。

四诊:诸症基本消除,仍偶有头昏,血压、血脂多次复查均正常,体重下降 4.5 kg。仍拟原法巩固治疗,处方:天麻10 g,菊花10 g,制何首乌12 g,枸杞子10 g,生山楂肉15 g,决明子10 g,泽泻15 g,炙白僵蚕10 g,荷叶15 g,桑寄生12 g,生牡蛎(先煎)30 g。

随访 3 个月,恙平未发,体重续有下降,患者极为满意,故治以黄精、何首乌、桑寄生培补肝肾;生山楂、丹参活血化瘀;白僵蚕、罗布麻叶、决明子等平肝潜阳熄风而奏效。滋肾养肝、化痰祛瘀乃周老多年经验的总结,实践证明具有良好效果,不仅降

高血压病的中医特色疗法

Luobumaye and Juemingzi for calming the liver, suppressing yang and wind. This therapeutic method of nourishing the kidney and liver, resolving phlegm and removing stasis has proved clinically to be effective in lowering blood-lipid, decreasing blood viscosity, reducing blood pressure and body weight, and significantly relieving the symptoms, enhancing constitution and delaying senility. In clinical practice, when prescription or drug is to be selected, the primary and secondary should be differentiated between the deficiency of the liver and kidney and the stagnation of phlegm and blood stasis; furthermore, complications should be considered.

Chapter Two   Jiao Shude's Experience

Section One   Understanding of Etiology and Pathogenesis

Jiao Shude, a senior doctor of TCM, believes that primary hypertension is related to "dizziness", "headache", "insomnia" and other diseases in TCM. In etiology and pathogenesis, its primary aspect is deficiency of the liver, kidney, heart and spleen, while the secondary is such pathogenic factors as wind, phlegm, qi and fire. It may result from the mutual influence between these

脂、降低血黏度、降压、减肥,而且可显著改善临床症状,增强体质,延缓衰老。临证尚需审辨肝肾不足与痰瘀阻滞的主次及兼夹症,进行处方选药。

二、焦树德治验

(一)病机新识

焦树德老中医认为高血压病与中医学"眩晕"、"头痛"、"失眠"等疾病相关。从病因病机来看,肝、肾、心、脾的正气虚为病之本,风、痰、气、火等邪气盛为病之标。标本互为因果,风、痰、气、火相兼为害,在一定条件下发病。从本虚方面来看,以肝阴

two aspects and combination of wind, phlegm, qi and fire in certain circumstances. In primary deficiency, deficiency of liver-yin, deficiency of both spleen and heart, and deficiency of kidney are mostly seen. Deficiency of liver-yin causes hyperactivity of liver-yang, resulting in stirring-up of liver-wind and disturbing-up of wind-yang. Deficiency of both the spleen and heart causes failure of qi and blood to nourish the brain, and deficiency of kidney causes insufficiency of spinal marrow, resulting in dizziness, tinnitus, blurred vision and weak lower limbs. Deficiency of the spleen in the middle-energizer causes failure of transformation and transportation and of clear-yang ascending, and causes upward disturbing of turbid phlegm, resulting in dizziness. In secondary excess, mental disorder, hyperactivity of heart-fire and liver-fire, overeating and overdrinking are mostly seen. Mental disorder, excessive joy or anger, worry, grief, fear and fright may impair the liver, kidney, heart and spleen, inducing upward disturbance of fire and wind phlegm, hyperactivity of liver-yang, or excessive heart-fire. Improper diet may damage the spleen and stomach and impair their transforming and transporting functions, changing middle-energizer into source of phlegm. However, the two aspects are closely related to each other and can change into each other in certain conditions. Their roles

不足,心脾血虚及肾虚较为常见。肝
阴不足则肝阳上亢,可使人肝风内
动,风阳上扰;心脾血虚则血不荣上,
气血不能上奉于脑;肾虚,髓海不足
则可使人脑转耳鸣,胫酸眩冒,目无
所见;脾虚中焦不化,清阳不升则可
致痰浊上犯,前人有"无痰不作眩"的
经验。从标实方面来看,以情志失
调,心肝火盛,暴饮暴食较常见。精
神因素失调,或过喜暴怒、忧思惊恐
等皆可以伤及肝肾心脾而导致化火、
生风、夹痰上扰,或肝阳过亢,或心火
暴甚等;饮食不节,伤害脾胃,致中运
不健则可成为生痰之源。当然标本
也不能截然分开,并且在疾病的不同
阶段,不同证候中又有主次先后的不
同,在一定时候也可以转化。一般看
来,在疾病初起阶段或青壮年患者,
常表现为邪盛、阳证,以标实为主。
在中期由于邪正斗争、标本转化等关
系,又可出现正虚邪实、本虚标实,或
上盛下虚等证。阴虚阳旺证是此时
期最常见的证候,后期则可以出现阴
阳俱虚,气血皆衰等证。

vary in different stages of the disease and with different syndromes. Generally, secondary excess is the main aspect of the disease in the early stage or among the young and middle-aged patients, manifested as pathogenic excess or yang syndrome. Syndromes as healthy-qi deficiency and pathogenic excess, primary deficiency and secondary excess, or excess in the upper and deficiency in the lower may appear later, due to the struggle between pathogenic factors and healthy-qi and transformation between the primary and the secondary aspect of the disease. In this stage yang hyperactivity and yin deficiency is the syndrome mostly seen, and in the advanced stage syndromes as deficiency of yin and yang, and exhaustion of qi and blood may be present.

Section Two   Diagnostic and Therapeutic Characteristics

1. Syndrome differentiation

Although primary hypertension may have many kinds of syndromes, the following four types are commonly seen in clinic, according to sufficiency or insufficiency of yin and yang, excess or deficiency of zang-fu organs, tongue coating, pulse condition, constitution, and predisposing factors.

(1) Hyperactivity of liver-yang: Mostly caused by

(二) 诊疗特色

1. 辨证论治

高血压病的临床证候很多，根据体内阴阳盛衰、脏腑虚实、舌苔、脉象、体型以及发病诱因等的不同，进行分析归纳，最常见的可有以下四种不同证型。

(1) 肝阳上亢：多由素体阳盛，

protracted sthenic yang, or by rage generating liver-fire, or by qi stagnation eliciting fire. Since yang represents moving and ascending, liver-yang disturbs upwards and liver-heat induces wind, so that the seven orifices are disturbed, resulting in primary hypertension.

Chief manifestations: Headache, dizziness, head distension, conjunctival congestion, flushed face, irritability, bitter taste in the mouth, constipation, darkish yellow urine, yellow tongue coating, and wiry and rapid pulse.

Therapeutic principle: Cool the blood and purge fire, calm the liver and suppress wind.

Prescription: Modified Longdan Xiegan Tang (decoction), composed of Longdancao, Huangqin, Shanzhizi, Xiakucao, Shengdaizheshi, Zexie, Cheqianzi, Caojueming, Kudingcha, Cijili and Chishaoyao. Increase the dosage of Longdancao, Huangqin, Shanzhi, Xiakucao, Shengzheshi and Zexie for excessive liver-fire; add Xiangfu, Qingpi, Chuanhoupo, Yujin and Baimeihua for qi stagnation; add Shengbaishao, Shengdihuang, Xuanshen and Shengshijueming for yin deficiency.

(2) Hyperactivity of liver with yin deficiency: Mostly caused by protracted deficient yin, or prolonged stress impairing yin, or prolonged illness consuming yin, there appear deficiency of liver-yin and kidney-yin, hyperactivity of liver-yang and internal disturbance of liver-wind,

或怒动肝火,或气郁化火致使肝阳亢盛。阳主动,主升,肝阳上冲,肝热生风,清窍受扰而致发病。

【主要证候】 头痛,头晕,头胀,目赤面红,急躁易怒,口苦便秘,尿黄赤。舌苔黄,脉弦数有力。

【治法】 苦寒直折,凉血泻火,平肝熄风。方选龙胆泻肝汤加减。

【处方】 龙胆草、黄芩、山栀子、夏枯草、生代赭石、泽泻、车前子、草决明、苦丁茶、刺蒺藜、赤芍药。肝火盛者,重用龙胆草、黄芩、山栀子、生代赭石、泽泻;气郁者,加香附、青皮、川厚朴、郁金、白梅花。兼有阴虚者,加生白芍药、生地黄、玄参、生石决明。

(2)阴虚肝旺:多由平素阴虚,或久劳伤阴,或久病耗阴等导致肝肾阴虚,肝阳偏旺,肝风内动而发病。

resulting in hypertension.

Chief manifestations: Dizziness, blurred vision, feeling of heaviness over the head, hemicrania, irritability, insomnia, dreaminess, feverish sensation of face, hand tremble, feverish sensation of palms in the afternoon, dry mouth in the afternoon and at night, red tongue with thin and white or yellow coating or without coating, and thready and rapid pulse.

Therapeutic principle: Nourish yin and suppress yang, soothe the liver and suppress wind.

Prescription: Modified Tianma Gouteng Yin (decoction), composed of Shengdihuang, Shengbaishaoyao, Xuanshen, Shengshijueming (decocted first), Shengmuli (decocted first), Shengdaizheshi (decocted first), Tianma, Gouteng, Sangjisheng, Niuxi, Xiakucao and Juhua. Remove Xiakucao and add Heshouwu, Nüzhenzi and Digupi instead for weak chi-pulse, weak lumbus and knees; remove Xuanshen and Juhua and add Lingcishi (decocted first), Shanzhuyu, Duzhong and Zexie for dizziness.

(3) Insufficiency of kidney essence: Mostly caused by congenital weakness with deficiency of kidney essence, or by excessive sexual activity impairing kidney and consuming kidney essence. Since the kidney controls marrow and the brain is the reservoir of marrow, "if reservoir be-

【主要证候】 头晕目花,头重脚轻,或偏头痛,烦躁易怒,失眠多梦,或面部阵阵轰热,或两手颤抖,午后手心发热,午后及夜间口干。舌质红,苔薄白、薄黄或无苔,脉象细数。

【治法】 养阴潜阳,柔肝熄风。方选天麻钩藤饮加减。

【处方】 生地黄、生白芍药、玄参、生石决明(先煎)、生牡蛎(先煎)、生代赭石(先煎)、天麻、钩藤、桑寄生、牛膝、夏枯草、菊花。尺脉沉弱,腰膝酸软者,去夏枯草,加何首乌、女贞子、地骨皮;头晕目眩,头重脚轻明显,两足无根者,去玄参、菊花,加灵磁石(先煎)、山茱萸、杜仲、泽泻。

(3)肾精亏虚:多由先天不足,肾精不充,或房劳伤肾,肾精亏耗而致。肾主髓,脑为髓海,"髓海不足,则脑转耳鸣"。另一方面,肾虚不能养肝,则肝阳易动,虚风上扰。

comes insufficient, vertigo and tinnitus will result". On the other hand, the deficient kidney failing to nourish the liver causes hyperactivity of liver yang and stirring-up of deficient wind.

Chief manifestations: Dizziness, blurred vision, headache with hollow sensation, tinnitus, hypomnesis, weak lumbus and legs, spiritlessness, red tongue, and sunken and thready pulse with weakness of chi pulse.

Therapeutic principle: Nourish the kidney and benefit essence, nourish the liver and suppress wind.

Prescription: Modified Qiju Dihuang Tang (decoction), composed of Shengdihuang, Shudihuang, Shanzhuyu, Shanyao, Zexie, Mudanpi, Fuling, Gouqizi, Juhua, Shayuanzi, Cijili, Niuxi and Gouteng. Add Digupi, Qinpi, Biejia and Guibanjiao for kidney-yin deficiency with feverish sensation in chest, palms and soles, thirst, nocturnal emission, and thready and rapid pulse. Add Rougui, Ziheche Powder (in divided doses), Yinyanghuo, and Chenxiang Powder (in divided doses) for kidney-yang deficiency with aversion to cold, impotence, cool sensation below lumbus, pain in heels, pale tongue, even-soft and weak pulse.

For climacteric hypertensive women with yin deficiency symptoms such as feverish sensation in chest, palms and soles, hot sensation of face, and thready

【主要证候】 头晕,目花,头部空痛,脑转耳鸣,记忆减退,腰腿酸软,精神委靡,不能耐劳。舌质红,脉沉细,两尺弱。

【治法】 滋肾填精,养肝熄风。杞菊地黄汤加减。

【处方】 生地黄、熟地黄、山茱萸、山药、泽泻、牡丹皮、茯苓、枸杞子、菊花、沙苑子、刺蒺藜、牛膝、钩藤。偏于肾阴虚者,兼见五心烦热,口渴梦遗,脉象细数,酌加地骨皮、秦皮、鳖甲、龟版胶等。偏于肾阳虚者,兼见畏寒阳痿,腰以下发凉,足跟痛,两腿无根,舌质淡,脉缓弱,酌加肉桂、紫河车粉(分冲)、淫羊藿、沉香粉(分冲)。

妇女更年期高血压病,表现为阴阳俱虚证者,既有五心烦热,面部烘热,烦躁,脉细等阴虚症,又有畏冷足

pulse, as well as yang deficiency symptoms such as aversion to cold, cold feet, sore lumbus and legs, and preference for warm, modified Erxian Tang (decoction) should be used, which is composed of Xianmao, Xianlingpi, Danggui, Bajitian, Huangbai, Zhimu, Niuxi, Shengdihuang, Shudihuang and Sangjisheng.

(4) Stirring-up of turbid phlegm: Obesity, or indulgence in fat and sweet food impairing the spleen and stomach causes accumulation of dampness in middle-energizer, leading to production of phlegm. The accumulation of the phlegm causes the stagnation of the spleen and liver, resulting in upward disturbance of liver wind and phlegm. On the other hand, turbid phlegm attacks the meridians and blocks the circulation of qi and blood, resulting in numbness of limbs and hemiplegia.

Chief manifestations: Distending and heavy sensation of head, dizziness, oppressed feeling in the chest and stomach, vomiting, poor appetite, sleepiness, white and greasy tongue coating, and wiry and smooth pulse.

Therapeutic principle: Dissipate turbid phlegm, benefit the liver and invigorate the spleen.

Prescription: Modified Xuanzhe Ditan Tang (decoction), composed of Xuanfuhua, Daizheshi, Banxia, Juhong, Zhishi, Zhuru, Fuling, Huangqin, Binlang, Gualou, Nanxing, Tianma and Gouteng. Remove Zhishi,

寒,腰腿酸痛,喜暖等阳虚症,可用二仙汤加减。处方如:仙茅、仙灵脾、当归、巴戟天、黄柏、知母、牛膝、生地黄、熟地黄、桑寄生等。

(4)痰浊上犯:素体肥胖或恣食肥甘,伤于脾胃,中湿不化,湿聚生痰,痰浊壅盛,脾壅肝郁,可致肝风挟痰上扰而发病。另一方面,痰浊流注经络,影响气血运行,亦可致肢体麻木,半身不遂等。

【主要证候】 头胀头重,如裹如蒙,眩晕且痛,胸膈满闷,呕恶痰涎,少食多寐。舌苔白腻,脉象弦滑。

【治法】 化痰降浊,调肝健脾。方选旋赭涤痰汤加减。

【处方】 旋覆花、代赭石、半夏、橘红、枳实、竹茹、茯苓、黄芩、槟榔、瓜蒌、南星、天麻、钩藤。大便溏薄,脉濡者,去枳实、黄芩、瓜蒌,加白术、

Huangqin, Gualou and add Baizhu, Caokouren and Chaoyiyiren for loose stool and soft pulse; remove Banxia and Nanxing and add Zhuli and Dannanxing for pathogenic fire elicited by phlegm stagnation.

The above four types of syndromes are often seen clinically and usually combine together. They influence each other and transform into each other under certain conditions. Therefore, the therapeutic principle should be applied in a flexible way.

2. Personal experience

(1) Hypertension is mostly manifested as the following syndromes, i. e. hyperactivity of liver-yang, liver hyperactivity with yin-deficiency and upward disturbance of wind-phlegm. So there have been such sayings as "endogenous wind syndromes manifested as convulsion and vertigo, etc. , all pertain to the liver ", "no fire, no phlegm moving; no phlegm, no dizziness" and "no phlegm, no dizziness, fire moves phlegm", which are valuable references in clinic. However, excess syndrome may change into deficiency syndrome, and deficiency syndrome can be mixed with excess. So attention should be paid to the mutual transformation between different syndromes. The excess mostly belongs to the secondary, deficiency usually pertains to the primary, the secondary comes from the primary, thus it is important to treat the weakness of

草蔻仁、炒薏苡仁等；痰郁化火者，去半夏，加竹沥，改南星为胆南星。

以上四种证候较为常见，临床上四证又常混合兼见，并且四者互为影响，在一定条件下，又可相互转化，故临证时必须灵活运用。

2. 几点体会

（1）高血压病以肝阳上亢，阴虚肝旺及风痰上扰证较为多见：所以前人有"诸风掉眩，皆属于肝"，"无火不动痰，无痰不生晕"及"无痰不作眩，痰因火动"等说。证之临床，确有参考价值。同时，要注意疾病的转化，实证可以转虚，虚证也可以挟实。实证多言其标，虚证多言其本，标是由本而生，故治疗时又要注意治本，抓住适当时机，治疗其正虚的一面。《内经》中有"上虚则眩"及"上气不足，脑为之不满，耳为之苦鸣，头为之苦倾，目为之眩"的说法；明代张景岳有"无虚不作眩"之论，足资参证。但是也要时时注意不可忽略实证的治

healthy qi timely. *Huangdi Canon of Medicine* says "deficiency in the upper part results in dizziness" and "qi deficiency in the head causes ringing ears, uncomfortable head, and dim eyes "; Zhang Jingyue in the Ming Dynasty pointed out that "no deficiency, no dizziness". In fact these viewpoints are practicable, but the treatment for the excess syndrome should never be neglected and even be applied first sometimes. For example, dizziness in Shaoyang and in Yangming diseases are of the excess syndrome; "dizziness due to phlegm retention in epigastrium, fullness in the chest and epigastrium", and dizziness caused by dampness stagnation, belong to excess syndrome, too. They should not be treated by invigoration. On the other hand, it must be noticed that various pathologic aspects including the secondary, the primary, deficiency, excess, wind, phlegm, qi, and fire are often mixed with each other. In hypertension, there exist common pathogeneses such as liver-yang hyperactivity, wind-phlegm upward disturbance and excess in the upper and deficiency in the lower, but different patients have different pathological characteristics, which needs careful analysis. Furthermore, it is important to differentiate the pathological aspects such as liver-wind, liver-yang, kidney deficiency, liver hyperfunction, phlegm blocking meridians, and upward disturbance of wind-phlegm, and to

疗,甚至有时必须先治其实。如少阳病之目眩、阳明病之眩冒,皆属实证;又如"心下有痰饮,胸胁支满,目眩"及湿郁之头眩,皆不能言虚,俱不可用补,应全面看问题,不可偏执。另一方面,标、本、虚、实、风、痰、气、火等又常兼杂并见,不可不知。高血压病,有其肝阳旺盛、风痰上扰、下虚上实等共性,但更重要的是要注意分析每个病人的特性,对肝风、肝阳、肾虚、肝旺、痰塞经络、风痰上扰等等,孰先孰后,主次标本,比重多少;缓急轻重,都须分辨清楚。立法组方,必须权衡准确,才能取得良好效果,千万不可用"对号入座"式的方法,生搬硬套。

make clear which is the primary and which is the secondary, so as to work out a therapy and a prescription accordingly. The therapeutic principle should not be applied mechanically, but with a certain degree of flexibility according to individual condition.

(2) Experience of the past generations may serve as references for clinical practice, for instance, "excess in the upper is treated with Jiudahuang, deficiency in the lower with Lurong wine", "to nourish the upper, by replenishing the root first", "treating the kidney is treating the liver, for both organs share the same origin", "treating the liver means suppressing wind, suppressing wind means purging fire, and purging fire means resolving phlegm", etc. However, it is better to combine these experience with the result of modern pharmaceutical study. Many herbal drugs are reported effective for blood pressure reduction, i. e. Sangjisheng, Duzhong, Yinyanghuo, Xuanshen, Shanzhuyu, Shanzhizi, Cijili, Gouteng, Shijueming, Xiakucao, Yejuhua, Sangbaipi, Dilong, Fuling, Banxia, Zexie, Niuxi, Gegen, Sangzhi, Gouqizi, Danshen, etc. which should be used on the basis of syndrome differentiation.

(3) Some drugs are used for particular purposes. Jingjie or Jingjiesui is used for protracted headache or migraine (the former for mild cases, the latter for serious

（2）前人的治疗经验对临床多有帮助：如："上实者治以酒大黄，上虚者治以鹿茸酒"，"欲荣其上，必灌其根"，"乙癸同源，治肾即治肝"，"治肝即熄风，熄风即降火，降火即所以治痰"等等，均可参考应用。在运用前人经验的同时，也要随时吸取近人的研究成果，如近代报道有降血压作用的中药：桑寄生、杜仲、淫羊藿、玄参、山茱萸、山栀子、刺蒺藜、钩藤、石决明、夏枯草、野菊花、桑白皮、地龙、茯苓、半夏、泽泻、牛膝、葛根、桑枝、枸杞子、丹参等，均可结合辨证选用。

（3）辨病用药：在治疗比较顽固的头痛、偏头痛时，常在辨证论治的应证方剂内，加用一些荆芥或荆芥穗

ones), because it can not only enter the blood (to which protracted headache is closely associated), lead other drugs to the head, but also disperse stagnated heat and clear the head. Headache can be relieved when qi and blood run smoothly through the head. Therefore when Jingjie (or Jingjiesui) is added for hypertension with headache, it always produces remarkable effect. Zexie (or combined with Digupi) is usually added for excessive liver-yang, for it can purge stagnated heat in liver meridian (in ancient times called the ministerial fire of the liver), leading the heat out of the body through urination. In the case of liver-heat stagnation associated with failure of kidney-yin to restrain liver-yang (in ancient times called failure of kidney-water to restrain liver-fire), Digupi should be added for clearing away heat and invigorating the kidney. When combined, the two drugs are significantly effective for purging the liver and nourishing the kidney.

(4) Primary hypertension can not be cured at one night, for it usually progresses gradually and lasts for a long period of time, so patience is needed in the treatment. At the same time, a close attention should be paid to its pathologic changes and therapeutic method or prescription should be used for a relatively long time. The chief drug such as Gouteng should be used in a large

（病情较轻者用荆芥，重者用荆芥穗），往往取得良效。因为荆芥（荆芥穗）既可兼入血分（头痛久者多与血分有关），又可引方内其他药力上达头部而发挥效果，还可疏散郁热而清头目。头部气血疏畅不滞则疼痛可减。故在治高血压病头痛明显者也常在辨证论治的基础上加用此品，对解决头痛有效。对属于肝阳旺的高血压病，常在辨证论治的方剂中加用泽泻，或与地骨皮同用。因为泽泻能泻肝经郁热（古称肝经相火），使邪热下行而出，肝经郁热不解者，又常有肾阴不能制肝阳之证（古人称肾水不能制相火），故又可配加地骨皮清热益肾，两药合用泻肝益肾，常取得相得益彰的效果。

（4）治疗高血压病不可求之过急：因本病多是渐积而来，祛病亦如抽丝，须逐步认识，连续观察，深入治疗，故在诊治过程中，要注意守法守方，坚持一段时间，以观后效。有些主要药物，药量宜稍重，例如用钩藤，不但药量须较大，而且要注意煎药时

dosage and "decocted later". Some drugs such as Sheng-daizheshi, Shengshijueming, Shengmuli and Lingcishi should be used in large dosage and decocted first for 10 – 15 minutes.

（5）Blood pressure sometimes can be lowered during the time when drugs are taken, but relapse soon after drugs are not taken. In this case, the treatment should be continued on the basis of syndrome differentiation. If the treatment focuses on the primary cause of the disease, the general condition of the patient will be progressively improved and blood pressure will be gradually stabilized. In fact, blood pressure will fluctuate sometimes, but that doesn't mean the treatment is ineffective, and it is unadvisable to give up the treatment.

（6）Since the body is an organic whole, attention should be paid to the causative treatment. Generally speaking, symptoms belong to the secondary, while pathogenic factors pertain to the primary. Blood pressure elevation and various clinical manifestations are "the secondary". While yinyang disorder in zangfu organs is "the primary", which causes blood pressure elevation and abnormal pulse, tongue and complexion. Hence, in the treatment of hypertension, TCM lays emphasis mainly on regulating yinyang balance of the whole body, rather than lowering blood pressure alone. Furthermore, the

"后下",久煎则效果不好。生代赭石、生石决明、生牡蛎、灵磁石等药量须重用,并要先下,待其煎煮 10～15 分钟后,再下他药。

(5)辨证求准,疗程要足:如遇到服药则有效,血压可降至正常,但停药一段时间,血压又回升的情况,要继续给予辨证论治,深入观察,循症求因,遵照治病必求其本的精神,进行治疗,则会一次比一次稳定的时间长,并且在全身情况都好转的基础上血压也就渐渐稳定。不要一见波动,即认为无效而放弃治疗。

(6)中医从整体观念出发,在治病时要求注意求本:临床上一般是以症状为标,病因为本。故认为高血压病的血压升高和各种自觉症状都是临床表现,是病之"标";导致产生自觉症状和血压升高以及引起脉象、舌诊、气色等出现异常的内脏阴阳盛衰的失调(失去动态平衡)是病之"本"。所以中医治疗高血压病,其着眼点是放在调整人体内阴阳的失调方面,而不是专注意降血压。但标本是相对

secondary and the primary of the disease are relative and tend to mutually transform, and the pathological nature varies within different stages of the disease. So, sometimes both the primary and the secondary are treated simultaneously, and sometimes the secondary is even treated prior to the primary. However, the ultimate aim of treatment is to benefit the primary and causative treatment should always be kept in mind in the treatment of hypertension.

Section Three   Typical Cases

1. Li, female, aged 40, worker.

The patient had suffered from dizziness and headache for more than 10 years since 1965, accompanied by blurred vision. BP: 23.9 -25.3/14.6 -16 kPa. She was diagnosed previously as primary hypertension and had taken Chinese and western medicines, but the effect was not obvious.

First visit (June 22, 1979): She experienced dizziness, pain of the temple and nape. Since the Spring Festival the year before, she had experienced numbness of left side of the body, distending sensation and limited motion of the right upper limb, which slightly alleviated somewhat by passive motion. Her stool was dry, urination and menstruation normal. She also told that she once suffered

的,又是可以转化的,故根据证情的不同或不同阶段的变化,也有时标本同治,甚至先治标再治本等等,而治标的目的最终还是要达到"治病必求其本"的要求。所以中医在诊治高血压病时要时时注意求本。

（三）验案举隅

1. 李某某,女,40岁,工人。

头晕头痛10余年。病始于1965年,自觉头晕而痛,并伴眼花。血压常在23.9～25.3/14.6～16 kPa之间波动。其他医院诊断为高血压病,曾服中西药治疗,效果不明显。于1979年6月22日来院诊治。

现感头晕头痛,以两侧及头项部为重。从去年春节以来,左半身麻木,左手发胀,甚则左上肢活动不利,被动活动后可稍缓解。大便干燥,小便如常,月经尚调。12年前有过浮肿。其母有高血压病。检查:心肺无异常,尿常规正常,眼底动脉硬化,脉

高血压病的中医特色疗法

from edema 12 years ago, and her mother had primary hypertension. Examination revealed ocular fundus arteriosclerosis, red tip of the tongue with thin and yellow coating, sunken, smooth and wiry pulse, which was slightly larger on the right-hand side, BP: 23.9/14.6 kPa. Examination of the heart and lung revealed nothing abnormal and routine urine examination showed normal.

Syndrome differentiation: Chronic retention of excessive endogenous dampness causes stagnation of phlegm, which generates heat and consumes yin, resulting in deficiency of yin and hyperactivity of yang. In this case, liver-wind and phlegm disturb upwards, resulting in dizziness, headache, red tip of the tongue with thin and yellow coating, and sunken, smooth and wiry pulse. The sunken and smooth pulse indicates the presence of phlegm, and the wiry pulse reflects the stirring-up of liver-wind complicated by phlegm. The right pulse is stronger than the left one, indicating that dampness in middle-energizer accumulates and further transforms into phlegm, which blocks the meridians and causes symptoms such as numbness and fullness of the extremities or even limited motion. Based on the comprehensive analysis of the data obtained by four diagnostic methods, this case is diagnosed as dizziness due to liver-yang hyperactivity, liver-wind stirring inside, and wind-phlegm disturbing up-

象沉滑弦,右脉大于左脉,舌尖红,苔薄黄,血压 23.9/14.6 kPa。

【辨证】　素体湿盛,湿郁生痰,痰郁日久,化热伤阴,阴虚阳亢,致肝风挟痰上扰,而见头晕头痛,舌尖红,苔薄黄,脉象沉滑,主内有痰浊。其脉弦,知有肝风挟痰上扰之势。右手脉象大于左手,知中湿不化。积湿成痰,痰阻经络,血脉不通,则肢体麻木发胀,甚至活动不利。四诊合参,诊为肝阳偏旺,肝风内动,风痰上扰,发为眩晕之证。

wards.

Therapeutic principle: Calm the liver, suppress yang, clear away heat and resolve phlegm, and supplemented by promoting blood circulation and activating meridians.

Prescription: Shengdaizheshi (decocted first) 30 g, Shengmuli (decocted first) 30 g, Shengshijueming (decocted first) 30 g, Niuxi 10 g, Cijili 10 g, Huangqin 10 g, Huajuhong 12 g, Banxia 10 g, Fuling 12 g, Xiangfu 10 g, Dannanxing 9 g, Quangualou 30 g, Jingjiesui 7 g, Chishaoyao 20 g and Honghua 9 g.

In the prescription, Daizheshi, Muli and Shijueming are used for calming the liver, suppressing yang and nourishing liver-yin; Cijili, Huangqin, Gualou, Niuxi and Jingjiesui for clearing away heat, dispersing fire and purging ascending wind-heat; Juhong, Banxia, Dannanxing, Gualou and Fuling for dissipating turbid phlegm; Dannanxing and Gualou for counteracting the warm property of Juhong and Banxia; Xiangfu and Huangqin for soothing the liver and clearing away heat; Honghua and Chishao for promoting blood circulation and activating meridians to suppress wind.

Second visit (July 3, 1979): After taking 10 doses of the above decoction, she experienced slight alleviation of all symptoms and had a smooth bowel movement. Her

【治法】 平肝潜阳,化痰清热,佐以活血通络。

【处方】 生代赭石(先煎)30 g,生牡蛎(先煎)30 g,生石决明(先煎)30 g,牛膝10 g,刺蒺藜10 g,黄芩10 g,化橘红12 g,半夏10 g,茯苓12 g,香附10 g,胆南星9 g,全瓜蒌30 g,荆芥穗7 g,赤芍药20 g,红花9 g。

方用代赭石、牡蛎、石决明平肝潜阳,兼益肝阴,配刺蒺藜、黄芩、瓜蒌、牛膝、荆芥穗清热降火,以熄风热上升之势;橘红、半夏、胆南星、瓜蒌、茯苓伍用,以化痰浊,恐橘红、半夏温燥故配以胆南星、瓜蒌;香附配黄芩可舒肝清郁热;佐以红花配赤芍药以行血活络,同时亦寓有血行风自灭之义。

7月3日二诊:服上药10剂,诸症稍减,大便通畅,脉苔同前,血压20/14 kPa,继投上方加地骨皮12 g,

pulse and tongue coating unchanged. BP: 20/14 kPa.
Add Digupi 12 g and Xuanshen 15 g to the previous prescription to help clearing away heat and subsiding fire.

Third visit (July 10, 1979): Dizziness and headache
were relieved, but neck rigidity still existed. Two tablets
of Fufang Jiang-ya Pian (tablet) were taken on July 5 and
7 respectively, BP: 17.3/10.6 kPa (BP did not reduce to
normal level even taking 6 tablets daily before). The
same decoction was prescribed and taking of Fufang
Jiangya Pian (tablet) stopped.

The patient no longer took Fufang Jiangya Pian (tablet) since August. Her condition had been stabilized. BP:
around 16/10.6 kPa. She kept on the treatment with Chinese herbal medicines. The prescription was composed of
Shengdaizheshi (decocted first) 30 g, Shengmuli (decocted first) 30 g, Shengshijueming (decocted first) 30 g,
Cijili 12 g, Huangqin 10 g, Juhong 10 g, Banxia 10 g,
Fuling 20 g, Xiangfu 10 g, Gualou 30 g, Zexie 12 g, Jingjie
10 g, Baishaoyao 12 g, Sangzhi 30 g and Digupi 12 g.

Follow-up (Sept. 18): No recurrence was observed
and BP remained 16/10.6 kPa.

2. Li, female, aged 41, worker.

First visit: Aug. 31, 1979.

The patient had a history of primary hypertension.
Five days ago, she experienced a sudden chest distress

玄参15 g,助其清降之力。

7月10日三诊:头晕头痛俱减,但自觉颈项尚发硬,故病家5日、7日各服复方降压片2片,今日血压17.3/10.6 kPa(以往每日服复方降压片6片,血压仍不能降至正常)。效不更方,守方继服,并嘱不要再服降压片。

自8月起,患者未再服复方降压片,病情稳定,血压维持在16/10.6 kPa,坚持服中药巩固疗效。处方:生代赭石(先煎)30 g,生牡蛎(先煎)30 g,生石决明(先煎)30 g,刺蒺藜12 g,黄芩10 g,橘红10 g,半夏10 g,茯苓20 g,香附10 g,瓜蒌30 g,泽泻12 g,荆芥10 g,白芍药12 g,桑枝30 g,地骨皮12 g。

9月18日随访,血压一直稳定在16/10.6 kPa。

2. 李某某,女,41岁,工人。1979年8月31日初诊。

既往有高血压病史。5天前在洗衣服时,突感憋气胸堵,继而面色紫

followed by facial cyanosis, vomiting of foam, loss of consciousness and urinary incontinence when washing clothes, and was sent to the emergency department. After proper treatment she was discharged with marked improvement. She wanted to take herbal medicines and came to see the doctor.

Present symptoms: Dizziness, blurred vision, preference for closing eyes, nausea, poor appetite, vague pain in the lower abdomen, and unsmooth bowel movement. Examination: Cooperation in the examination, clear speech, sleepiness, dizziness and nausea whenever sitting up, eyes closed, spiritlessness, overweight, limbs movable freely, heart and lung normal, abdomen soft, spleen and liver impalpable, pulse sunken, thready and smooth, tongue coating white. BP: 25.3/14.6 kPa.

Syndrome differentiation: Overweight, white tongue coating, and smooth pulse were the signs of excess of internal turbid phlegm; dizziness and blurred vision indicated stirring-up of liver wind. Wind-phlegm disturbing upward resulted in dizziness and nausea. Incoordination between the liver and spleen caused the impaired function of transformation and transportation, resulting in unsmooth bowel movement. Based on the analysis of all symptoms and signs, it was diagnosed as a syndrome of excess of turbid phlegm and stirring-up of liver-wind.

Typical TCM Therapy for Primary Hypertension

青,口吐白沫,不省人事,小便失禁。经本院急诊室诊治,现已好转,因愿服中药,前来就医。

现感头晕目眩,两眼喜闭,恶心欲吐,不思饮食,有时少腹隐痛,大便不畅。检查:神情合作,言语清晰,嗜卧不起,起则头晕欲呕,目闭无神,体型较胖,四肢活动自如,心肺未见异常,腹软,肝脾未及,血压25.3/14.6 kPa,脉沉细滑,舌苔白。

【辨证】　体胖、苔白、恶心、脉滑乃痰浊内壅之征,头晕、目眩为肝风内动之象。风痰上扰,胃失和降,故眩晕欲吐。肝脾失和,中运不健,故大便不畅。综观脉症,诊为痰浊壅盛,肝郁风动之证。

高血压病的中医特色疗法

Therapeutic principle: Resolve phlegm and lower the adverse qi, calm the liver and expel wind, and supplemented by regulating the spleen and stomach.

Prescription: Banxia 10 g, Huajuhong 12 g, Fuling 12 g, Zhinanxing 10 g, Zhuru 10 g, Zexie 12 g, Gouteng 30 g (decocted first), Lingcishi (decocted first) 20 g, Zhenzhumu (decocted first) 30 g, Shengxiangfu 12 g, Jiaobinlang 10 g, and Sangjisheng 25 g, together with Muxiang Binglang Wan (pill) 5 g, twice daily.

Second visit (Sept. 4, 1979): The patient felt that dizziness and blurred vision was alleviated, spirit and appetite improved, able to open eyes and had a smooth bowel movement. Her pulse was sunken, thready, wiry and moderate, tongue coating thin and white, BP: 16/12 kPa. So the above prescription was modified by removing Binlang and Zhuru and adding Fangfeng 10 g and Cijili 12 g to enhance the effect of calming the liver and suppressing wind.

Third visit (Sept. 18): The patient had mild dizziness, left-side headache, feverish sensation in esophageal region, distending pain in the chest, and neck rigidity. Her pulse was sunken and wiry, tongue coating thin and white. BP: 17.3/12 kPa. So the second prescription was modified by removing Zexie, Sangjisheng, Cishi and Zhenzhumu, and adding Juhua 12 g, Huangqin 10 g, Gegen 20 g and Gualou 30 g.

【治法】　化痰降逆,平肝熄风,佐以和中。

【处方】　半夏10 g,化橘红12 g,茯苓12 g,制南星10 g,竹茹10 g,泽泻12 g,钩藤30 g(先煎)30 g,灵磁石(先煎)20 g,珍珠母(先煎)30 g,生香附12 g,焦槟榔10 g,桑寄生25 g。
另:木香槟榔丸5 g,每日2次。

9月4日二诊:药后头晕目眩减轻,大便通畅,眼已睁开,有神,食纳好转,脉沉细滑缓,舌苔薄白,血压16/12 kPa。上方去槟榔、竹茹,加防风10 g,刺蒺藜12 g,以加强平肝熄风之力。

9月18日三诊:尚感头晕,左偏头痛,自觉食管部发热,胸胀痛,项部发滞,脉沉滑,苔薄白,血压 17.3/12 kPa。二诊方去泽泻、桑寄生、磁石、珍珠母,加菊花12 g,黄芩10 g,葛根20 g,瓜蒌30 g。

Fourth visit (Sept. 25, 1979): Dizziness was markedly alleviated, headache totally relieved, blood pressure remained normal and lumbago occasionally appeared. Tongue coating and pulse unchanged. To invigorate the kidney and healthy qi, the third prescription was modified by removing Juhong and Fangfeng and adding Xuduan 15 g and Sangjisheng 25 g.

Chapter Three   Deng Tietao's Experience

Section One   Understanding of Etiology and Pathogenesis

Professor Deng Tietao, a senior TCM doctor, believes that according to its manifestations, hypertension is mainly caused by disorder of the liver. This organ shares the nature of wind and wood. The liver substance belongs to yin, while its function to yang. It is a rigid-natured organ, controlling moving and ascending. It can be impaired by emotional changes including anger and mental stress, causing hypertension with liver-yang hyperactivity. Hyperactive yang may develop gradually into pathogenic wind and fire and result in wind-stroke (cerebrovascular accident). The development of liver yang hyperactivity may also consume yin and impair the kidney, cau-

9月25日四诊：头晕显著减轻，头痛已除，血压一直正常，偶感腰痛，脉苔同前。予三诊方去橘红、防风，加续断15 g，桑寄生25 g，以益肾固本，巩固疗效。

三、邓铁涛治验

（一）病机新识

邓铁涛老中医认为，从高血压病的证候表现来看，其受病之脏主要属于肝的病变。肝为风木之脏，体阴用阳，其性刚，主动主升。情志失节，心情失畅，恼怒与精神紧张，都足以伤肝，可出现肝阳过亢的高血压，肝阳过亢继续发展，可以化风、化火而出现中风证候（脑血管意外）。肝阳过亢不已，可以伤阴伤肾，又进而出现阴阳两虚的证候。

sing yin and yang deficiency syndrome.

The kidney is closely related to the liver, and our ancestors compared the relationship between the kidney and the liver to that between the mother and the son. Kidney-yin deficiency may result from congenital insufficiency or daily life derangement. The insufficient yin may fail to nourish the liver and restrain liver-yang, and further cause hypertension of yang-hyperactivity and yin-deficiency type, which may also develop into hypertension or wind-stroke of yin-yang deficiency type later.

The heart may be damaged by extreme worry and the spleen be impaired by overstrain. Disorders of the heart and the spleen may result in pathologic changes in two ways. Firstly, it causes stagnation of the liver and obstruction of the spleen and upward disturbance of turbid phlegm. Secondly, it causes deficiency of spleen-yin, deficiency of blood nutrition, impairment of purifying and descending function of the lung, and sideways invasion of liver-qi. This kind of hypertension is usually associated with the heart and the spleen syndrome.

Section Two   Diagnostic and Therapeutic Characteristics

Professor Deng holds that this disease is closely related to the liver and regulation of the liver is the key in its

　　肝与肾的关系最为密切,前人用母(肾)与子(肝)形容两者的关系。先天不足或生活失节而致肝肾阴虚,肾阴不足不能涵木引致肝阳偏亢,出现阴虚阳亢之高血压。其发展亦可引起阴阳俱虚的高血压或中风等证。

　　忧思劳倦伤脾或劳心过度伤心,心脾受损,一方面可因痰浊上扰,土壅木郁,肝失条达而成高血压;一方面脾阴不足,血失濡养,肺失肃降,肝气横逆而成高血压。这一类高血压,往往兼见心脾之证。

(二) 诊疗特色

　　邓老认为本病与肝的关系至为密切,调肝为治疗高血压病的重要一

treatment. But it does not mean that the treatment is only confined to the drugs attributable to the liver meridian. In his book *Evening Talks in Xixi Study*, Wang Xugao in the Qing Dynasty summarized 30 kinds of therapeutic principles for regulating or counteracting liver-qi, liver-fire and liver-wind, and as well a great many drugs, which are still valuable for clinical use. Wang used to make the syndrome differentiation from the three aspects, i. e. liver-qi, liver-fire and liver-wind. Although he applied many therapeutic principles, he laid particular stress on nourishing yin. In fact, the syndromes of liver-qi, liver-fire and liver-wind are not always related to hypertension, but the physicians of later generations have accepted some of Wang's treatments. Ye Tianshi, another great physician in the same dynasty, had rich experience in treating such syndrome as "liver-wind". So in Ye Tianshi's medical records, Hua Xiuyun summarized Ye's experience in treating liver-wind under the term "liver-wind syndrome". In a word, regulating the liver is very important for treating hypertension. But its pathologic changes are complicated, hence the treatment must be based on the syndrome differentiation.

Hyperactivity of liver-yang should be treated by soothing the liver and suppressing yang with Shijue Muli Tang (decoction), which is composed of Shijueming (de-

环,但治肝不一定限于肝经之药。清代王旭高《西溪书屋夜话录》记载肝气、肝火、肝风的疗法共有 30 种,用药颇广,值得参考。王氏治肝,以肝气、肝火、肝风辨证。王氏治肝之法虽多,而偏重于清滋。肝气、肝风、肝火之证,不等于只属于高血压,但其中一些治法,已为后世所采用。清代医家叶天士早已对肝风一类病有较丰富的经验。如华岫云为叶天士医案立"肝风"一证,总结叶氏治肝风之法。治疗高血压,治肝是重要的一环,但疾病变化多端,不能执一,应辨证论治。

肝阳上亢证,宜平肝潜阳,用石决牡蛎汤:石决明(先煎)30 g,生牡蛎(先煎)30 g,白芍药15 g,牛膝15 g,

cocted first) 30 g, Shengmuli (decocted first) 30 g, Baishaoyao 15 g, Niuxi 15 g, Gouteng (decocted later) 15 g, Lianzixin 6 g, and Lianxu 10 g. In this prescription, Shijueming and Muli are principal drugs for calming the liver and suppressing yang; Gouteng and Baishaoyao are the assistant for suppressing liver-wind; Lianzixin and Lianxu are the adjuvant respectively for clearing the heart and soothing the liver and for nourishing the kidney and benefiting essence; Niuxi is the guide for sending drugs to descend. Add Huangqin for yellow tongue coating, rapid and strong pulse; add Dahuang for constipation; add Fuling and Zexie but remove Lianxu for thick and greasy tongue coating; add Juhua or Longdancao for serious headache of heat type; add Tianma for serious dizziness; add Yejiaoteng or Suanzaoren for insomnia.

Deficiency of liver-yin and kidney-yin should be treated by nourishing the liver and kidney with Lianshen Tang (decoction), which is composed of Lianxu 12 g, Sangshenzi 12 g, Nüzhenzi 12 g, Hanliancao 12 g, Shanyao 15 g, Guiban (decocted first) 30 g, and Niuxi 15 g. In this prescription, Lianxu, Sangshen, Nüzhenzi and Hanliancao are the principal drugs to nouish the liver and kidney; Shanyao, Guiban and Shengmuli are the assistant, and Niuxi is the guide. Add Taizishen for healthy-qi deficiency; add Maimendong and Shengdihuang for

钩藤（后下）15 g，莲子心6 g，莲须10 g。此方用介类之石决明、牡蛎以平肝潜阳为主药，钩藤、白芍药平肝熄风为辅药，莲子心清心平肝，莲须益肾固精为佐，牛膝下行为使药。如苔黄、脉数有力加黄芩；若兼阳明实热便秘者，可加大黄之类泻其实热；苔厚腻去莲须加茯苓、泽泻；头痛甚属热者加菊花或龙胆草；头晕甚加明天麻；失眠加夜交藤或酸枣仁。

肝肾阴虚证，宜滋肾养肝，用莲椹汤：莲须12 g，桑椹子12 g，女贞子12 g，旱莲草12 g，山药15 g，龟版（先煎）30 g，牛膝15 g。此方以莲须、桑椹、女贞子、旱莲草滋养肝肾为主药；山药、龟版、生牡蛎为辅药；牛膝为使药。气虚加太子参；舌光无苔加麦门冬、生地黄；失眠心悸加酸枣仁、柏子仁。

bald tongue, and add Suanzaoren and Baiziren for insomnia and palpitation.

For yin and yang deficiency, it should be treated by nourishing the liver and kidney and suppressing yang with Ganshen Shuangbu Tang (decoction), which is composed of Sangjisheng 30 g, Heshouwu 24 g, Chuanxiong 9 g, Yinyanghuo 9 g, Yumixu 30 g, Duzhong 9 g, Cishi (decocted first) 30 g, and Shenglonggu (decocted first) 30 g. Add Huangqi 30 g for healthy qi deficiency. In the case with chief manifestations of yang deficiency, Fugui Shiwei Tang (decoction) (Rougui 3 g, Shufuzi 10 g, Huangjing 20 g, Sangshen 10 g, Mudanpi 9 g, Yunfuling 10 g, Zexie 10 g, Lianxu 12 g, Yumixu 30 g, and Niuxi 9 g) should be used. For kidney-yang deficiency with edema, Zhenwu Tang (decoction) with additions of Huangqi 30 g and Duzhong 12 g should be used.

For qi deficiency and turbid phlegm syndrome, it should be treated by invigorating the spleen and nourishing qi with Zhejue Jiuwei Tang (decoction), which is composed of Huangqi 30 g, Dangshen 15 g, Chenpi 6 g, Fabanxia 12 g, Yunfuling 15 g, Daizheshi (decocted first) 30 g, Caojueming 24 g, Baizhu 9 g, and Gancao 2 g. In the prescription, Huangqin is used in large dosage and combined with drugs of Liujunzi Tang (decoction) to nourish qi and dissipate turbid phlegm; with Daizheshi

阴阳两虚证,宜补肝肾潜阳,方用肝肾双补汤:桑寄生30 g,何首乌24 g,川芎9 g,淫羊藿9 g,玉米须30 g,杜仲9 g,磁石(先煎)30 g,生龙骨(先煎)30 g。若兼气虚加黄芪30 g。若以肾阳虚为主者,用附桂十味汤(肉桂3 g,熟附子10 g,黄精20 g,桑椹10 g,牡丹皮9 g,云茯苓10 g,泽泻10 g,莲须12 g,玉米须30 g,牛膝9 g)。若肾阳虚甚兼浮肿者,用真武汤加黄芪30 g,杜仲12 g。

气虚痰浊证,宜健脾益气,用赭决九味汤:黄芪30 g,党参15 g,陈皮6 g,法半夏12 g,云茯苓15 g,代赭石(先煎)30 g,草决明24 g,白术9 g,甘草2 g。此方重用黄芪合六君子汤补气以除痰浊,配以代赭石、决明子以降逆平肝。若兼肝肾阴虚者加何首乌、桑椹、女贞子之属,若兼肾阳虚者加肉桂心、仙茅、淫羊藿之属,若兼血瘀

and Juemingzi to calm the liver and subside adverseness; add Heshouwu, Sangshen and Nüzhenzi for liver-yin and kidney-yin deficiency; add Rouguixin, Xianmao and Yin-yanghuo for kidney-yang deficiency; add Chuanxiong and Danshen for stagnation of blood.

In Deng's opinion, comprehensive measures based on the etiologic and pathogenic characteristics should be taken in the prevention and treatment for hypertension.

1. Regulation of emotional activity

Psychic factors and work stress are closely related to this disease, so it is important for the patient to have a nice psychic environment and a well-arranged work. Since internal causes are the decisive factor, psycho-therapy and a proper arrangement of work and rest are also important. What is more, a proper diet and life style should be taken into account.

2. Physical therapy

Many kinds of sports such as setting-up exercise and Taijiquan are effective measures to prevent and treat this disease.

3. Combination of Chinese and western medicine

Treatment combined by Chinese and western medi-cine is also necessary. Western medicines usually have a quick action, while Chinese herbal drugs have a slow but persistent action, so combination of both can be used

者加川芎、丹参之属。

邓老强调若从预防与比较系统彻底的治疗来说，应针对病因病机采取综合措施。

1. 调节情志

本病与精神因素，工作紧张关系较大，对患者的精神环境与工作安排十分重要。当然患者的内因是决定的因素，因此做好患者的思想工作与注意劳逸结合，是一个重要的措施。饮食与生活上的调节都很重要。

2. 体育疗法

各项体育运动如健身操、太极拳等，都是行之有效的方法。不论预防与治疗，都有可靠的作用。

3. 中西并用

中西结合治疗也是需要的，西药疗效快，中药疗效慢但比较巩固，可以因势结合使用。如见高血压危象，先用西药或针灸（针刺太冲穴用泻法

according to individual cases. Hypertensive crisis, for example, can first be treated by western drug or acupuncture (puncture at Taichong (LR 3) by reducing method) and then by both Chinese and western drugs. Intractable hypertension can also be treated with Chinese and western drugs, and then by Chinese drugs alone when the condition is stabilized.

Section Three   Typical Cases

Chen, male, aged 62, physician of TCM.

First visit: May 9, 1984.

Medical history: On the evening of May 8, 1984, his right extremities were weakened suddenly when the patient was having a shampoo, and soon became paralyzed. He was unable to speak and then lost consciousness. He was sent to the local health station and examination revealed that T 37.8℃, BP: 21.3/14.7 kPa, comatose and obese, posture passive, face flushed, pupils equal, nasolabial groove shallowed, mouth angle deviated toward the left, neck soft, lung emphysematous with tiny wet rale at the base, HR 104/min with irregular beats, right limbs paralyzed, Babinski's sign positive. He had primary hypertension for 10 years and was indulged in smoking and drinking. A consultation was once held with neurologists from nearby hospital, a non-identified diagnosis was

可治高血压危象）控制，然后中西并用。对顽固之高血压亦宜中西并用，至一定时期后才纯用中药。

（三）验案举隅

陈某，男，62 岁，中医师。初诊：1984 年 5 月 9 日。

病史：患者于 1984 年 5 月 8 日晚洗头时突觉右侧上下肢活动无力，继而出现失语，右侧上下肢体偏瘫，神志昏迷，即请当地卫生所值班医师检查，体温 37.8℃，血压 21.3/14.7 kPa，神志昏迷，被动体位，体胖，面赤身热，双瞳孔等圆等大，右鼻唇沟变浅，口角左歪，颈软，肺气肿征，双肺底可闻小湿啰音，心率 104 次/分，律不整，右侧上下肢体弛缓，巴彬斯基征阳性。既往有高血压病史 10 多年，平素嗜烟酒。起病后曾请附近医院神经科医师会诊，拟为"脑出血与脑血栓待定，建议暂不宜

made as "cerebral hemorrhage or embolism". He was advised not to be moved to anywhere until the condition became stabilized. Since this health station was not well-equipped and its facilities were limited, Dr. Deng was asked for consultation.

Examination: Besides the above symptoms, the patient was irritable, with occasional muscular contraction, breath coarse with foul smell, wheezing sound in the throat, no urination nor bowel movement, lips red and dry, tongue deep-red with yellow, thick and dry coating, pulse wiry, smooth and rapid.

Syndrome differentiation: Wind-stroke syndrome (directly attacking zangfu organs) attributable to stirring-up of liver-wind and phlegm-stagnation blocking orifices.

Therapeutic principle: Calm the liver and suppress wind, eliminate phlegm and remove stasis to induce resuscitation.

Prescription: a. Angong Niuhuang Wan (pill), one and a half pill daily, one swallowed with water, the half smashed and mixed with cool water (10 ml) and dipped on the tongue frequently. b. Puncture both sides of Taichong (LR3) with reducing method. c. Herbal medicine: Lingyangjiao 30 g (decocted first), Zhuru 12 g, Tianzhuhuang 5 g, Caojueming 20 g, Dannanxing 10 g, Dilong 10 g, Tianqipian (decocted first) 10 g, Juhong 10 g, Li-

搬动,应原地治疗,待病情稳定后再送医院作CT进一步确诊",因所在地为工厂卫生所,鉴于设备及医疗条件所限,治疗上颇感棘手,遂请邓老会诊。

【诊查】 症如上述,烦躁,间有抽筋,气粗口臭,喉间痰声辘辘,大小便闭,口唇红而干,舌红绛,苔黄厚干焦,脉弦滑数。

【辨证】 中风证(直中脏腑)。证属肝风内动,痰瘀阻塞清窍。

【治法】 平肝熄风,豁痰化瘀开窍。

【处方】 ① 安宫牛黄丸每日一粒半,其中一粒内服,余半粒用冷开水10 ml调匀,用棉签频频点舌。② 针泻太冲(双)。③ 中药:羚羊角(先煎)30 g,竹茹12 g,天竺黄5 g,草决明20 g,胆南星、地龙、田七片(先煎)、橘红各10 g,连翘12 g,陈皮5 g,丹参18 g,每日 1 剂,连服 4 日,第 2

anqiao 12 g, Chenpi 5 g, and Danshen 18 g. The patient was asked to take 4 doses of the decoction, one dose daily. On the 2nd day, complication of pulmonary infection occurred, penicillin, 800,000 U and streptomycin 1 g, im, twice daily for 1 week.

Second visit (May 13, 1984): The patient became conscious, with normal breathing. No wheezing sound was heard in the throat. Aphasia, hemiplegia and constipation remained unchanged. Bad smell lessened, red tongue with thick and yellow coating, pulse wiry and smooth. BP: 18/12 kPa.

Prescription: a. Angong Nuihuang Wan (pill), used in the same way as above. b. Dahuang 30 g, decocted with water to 200 ml, used for low retention-enema (one hour later, he defecated three times with a quantity about 1,000 ml). c. Herbal medicine: Shijueming 30 g (decocted first), Zhuru 12 g, Baishaoyao 15 g, Zhishi 10 g, Shichangpu 10 g, Dannanxing 10 g, Fabanxia 10 g, Tianqipian (decocted first) 10 g, Juluo 10 g, Danshen 10 g, and Taizishen 20 g, one dose daily for 4 days.

On May 17, he was sent to a hospital for CT examination, the result revealed a hematoma (about 5.5 cm × 3.5 cm × 6 cm) at the base of the left cerebral hemisphere and internal capsule. When the condition became stabilized, he was shifted to a TCM hospital on the same day.

日由于患者合并肺部感染较明显,故加强抗感染,肌注青霉素 80 万 U、链霉素 1 g,每日 2 次,连用 1 周。

二诊:5 月 13 日。患者神智转清,喉间痰鸣消失,呼吸平顺,口臭略减,失语及右侧上下肢偏瘫如前,大便自起病后闭结,舌红,苔黄厚干,脉弦滑。血压 18.7/12 kPa。

【处方】　① 安宫牛黄丸用法同前。② 大黄 30 g,煎水 200 ml 低位保留灌肠(灌肠后约 1 小时排便 3 次,量约 1 000 g)。③ 中药:石决明(先煎)30 g,竹茹 12 g,白芍药 15 g,枳实、石菖蒲、胆南星、法半夏、田七片(先煎)、橘络、丹参各 10 g,太子参 20 g,每日 1 剂,连服 4 日。

5 月 17 日外出到某医院作颅脑 CT 检查,意见为:大脑左半球底部和内囊部位血肿(大小约 5.5 cm×3.5 cm×6 cm)。因病情稳定,经家属要求于 5 月 17 日转某中医院住

During hospitalization, he was given Chinese and Western medicines such as Angong Niuhuan Wan (pill), Wendan Tang (decoction), Xingnaojing (injection) and energy mixture.

Third visit (June 6, 1984): The patient was conscious but tired, speech unclear, right limbs paralyzed, urination and defecation normal, tongue pale with thin coating, and pulse thready. Syndrome differentiation: Deficiency of qi and blood, and blockage of meridians. The therapeutic principle was invigorating qi and nourishing blood, removing blood-stasis and activating meridians.

Prescription: Modified Buyang Huanwu Tang (decoction), composed of Huangqi 100 g, Chishaoyao 6 g, Chuanxiong 6 g, Dangguiwei 6 g, Taoren 6 g, Honghua 6 g, Dilong 10 g, Shichangpu 10 g, Wuzhualong 30 g, and Jixueteng 30 g, one dose daily.

In addition, the patient took Houzhao San (powder), one vial daily. The above recipe was used as the basic prescription of recuperative treatment for one year.

CT reexamination (June 6, 1985) revealed that the hematoma in the left cerebral hemisphere was absorbed and the cavity formation was present.

The patient is still alive and able to take care of himself in daily life.

院。住院期间,中药用安宫牛黄丸、温胆汤,西药用能量合剂、醒脑净等。

三诊:6 月 6 日。神清,体倦神疲,语言不利,右侧肢体偏瘫,二便自调,舌质淡,苔薄白,脉细。证属气血两虚,脉络瘀阻。改用益气养血、祛瘀通络。拟方用补阳还五汤加味。

【处方】 黄芪100 g,赤芍药、川芎、当归尾、桃仁、红花各6 g,地龙、石菖蒲各10 g,五爪龙、鸡血藤各30 g,每日 1 剂。

另加服猴枣散早晚各 1 支,用上方为基本方加减作善后调治近 1 年。

1985 年 6 月 6 日颅脑 CT 复查意见为:大脑左半球血肿吸收后空洞形成。现患者仍健在。生活基本能自理。

Index

B

Baifan / *Alumen*

Baifuzi / *Rhizoma Typhonii*

Baihuasheshecao / *Herba Hedyotis Diffusae*

Baijiangcan / *Bombyx Batryticatus*

Baijiezi / *Semen Sinapis*

Baijili / *Fructus Tribuli*

Baijuhua / *Flos Chrysanthemi*

Baimeihua / *Flos Mume*

Baishaoyao / *Radix Paeoniae Alba*

Baizhi / *Radix Angelicae Dahuricae*

Baizhu / *Rhizoma Atractylodis Macrocephalae*

Baiziren / *Semen Platycladi*

Bajirou / *Epidermis Morindae Officinalis*

Bajitian / *Radix Morindae Officinalis*

Banxia / *Rhizoma Pinelliae*

Beimu / *Bulbus Fritillariae Cirrhosae*

Biejia / *Carapax Trionycis*

Bingpian / *Borneolum Syntheticum*

Binlang / *Semen Arecae*

Bohe / *Herba Menthae*

索　引

白矾

白附子

白花蛇舌草

白僵蚕

白芥子

白蒺藜

白菊花

白梅花

白芍药

白芷

白术

柏子仁

巴戟肉

巴戟天

半夏

贝母

鳖甲

冰片

槟榔

薄荷

高血压病的中医特色疗法

Buguzhi / *Fructus Psoraleae*

C

Cangzhu / *Rhizoma Atractylodis*

Caojueming / *Semen Cassiae*

Caokouren / *Semen Alpiniae Katsumadai*

Cebaiye / *Cacumen Platycladi*

Chaihu / *Radix Bupleuri*

Chantui / *Periostracum Cicadae*

Chaohuangqin / *Radix Scutellariae Preparata*

Chaoyiyiren / *Semen Coicis Preparata*

Chaozhimu / *Rhizoma Anemarrhenae Preparata*

Chendanxing / *Arisaema cum Bile*

Chenpi / *Pericarpium Citri Reticulatae*

Chenxiang / *Lignum Aquilariae Resinatum*

Cheqiancao / *Herba Plantaginis*

Cheqianzi / *Semen Plataginis*

Chishaoyao / *Radix Paeoniae Rubra*

Chongweizi / *Fructus Leonuri*

Chouwutong / *Folium Clerodendri Trichotomi*

Chuanduzhong / *Cortex Eucommiae*

Chuanlianzi / *Fructus Toosendan*

Chuanniuxi / *Radix Cyathulae*

Chuanhoupo / *Cortex Magnoliae Officinalis*

Chuanwu / *Radix Aconiti*

Chuanxiong / *Rhizoma Chuanxiong*

补骨脂

苍术
草决明
草蔻仁
侧柏叶
柴胡
蝉蜕
炒黄芩
炒薏苡仁
炒知母
陈胆星
陈皮
沉香
车前草
车前子
赤芍药
茺蔚子
臭梧桐
川杜仲
川楝子
川牛膝
川厚朴
川乌
川芎

高血压病的中医特色疗法

Cijili / *Fructus Tribuli*

Cishi / *Magnetitum*

D

Dahuang / *Radix et Rhizoma Rhei*

Daizheshi / *Haematitum*

Daji / *Herba seu Radix Cirsii Japonici*

Dancongrong / *Herba Cistanches*

Danfen / *Fel Ursi*

Danggui / *Radix Angelicae Sinensis*

Dangguiwei / *Lateralis Angelicae Sinensis Radix*

Dangguixu / *Fibra Angelicae Sinensis Radix*

Dangshen / *Radix Codonopsis*

Danhuangqin / *Radix Scutellariae*

Dannanxing / *Arisaema cum Bile*

Danshen / *Radix Salviae Miltiorrhizae*

Danzhuye / *Herba Lophatheri*

Dashengdihuang / *Radix Rehmanniae*

Dashudihuang / *Radix Rehmanniae Preparata*

Dazao / *Fructus Jujubae*

Digupi / *Cortex Lycii*

Dilong / *Pheretima*

Dongsangye / *Folium Mori*

Duzhong / *Cortex Eucommiae*

E

Ejiao / *Colla Corii Asini*

刺蒺藜

磁石

大黄

代赭石

大蓟

淡苁蓉

胆粉

当归

当归尾

当归须

党参

淡黄芩

胆南星

丹参

淡竹叶

大生地黄

大熟地黄

大枣

地骨皮

地龙

冬桑叶

杜仲

阿胶

高血压病的中医特色疗法

F

Fabanxia / *Rhizoma Pinelliae Preparata*

Fangfeng / *Radix Saposhnikoviae*

Fangji / *Radix Stephaniae Tetrandrae*

Fanyujin / *Radix Curcumae et Alumen*

Fenghuaxiao / *Natrii Sulfas*

Fuling / *Poria*

Fushen / *Sclerotium Poriae Circum Radicem Pini*

Fuzi / *Radix Aconiti Lateralis Preparata*

G

Gancao / *Radix Glycyrrhizae*

Gandihuang / *Radix Rehmanniae*

Gandilong / *Pheretima*

Gansui / *Radix Kansui*

Gegen / *Radix Puerariae*

Gouqizi / *Fructus Lycii*

Gouteng / *Ramulus Uncariae cum Uncis*

Gualou / *Fructus Trichosanthis*

Gualoupi / *Pericarpium Trichosanthis*

Guangdilong / *Pheretima*

Guiban / *Carapax et Plastrum Testudinis*

Guibanjiao / *Colla Carapais et Plastri Testudinis*

Guizhi / *Ramulus Cinnamomi*

H

Haizao / *Sargassum*

法半夏

防风

防己

矾郁金

风化硝

茯苓

茯神

附子

甘草

干地黄

干地龙

甘遂

葛根

枸杞子

钩藤

瓜蒌

瓜蒌皮

广地龙

龟版

龟版胶

桂枝

海藻

高血压病的中医特色疗法

Hanfangji / *Radix Stephaniae Tetrandrae*

Hanliancao / *Herba Ecliptae*

Hanqincai / *Herba Apii Graveolentis*

Heishanzhizi / *Fructus Gardeniae*

Heizhima / *Semen Sesami Nigrum*

Heshouwu / *Radix Polygoni Multiflori*

Heye / *Folium Nelumbinis*

Honghua / *Flos Carthama*

Hongzao / *Fructus Jujubae*

Houzao/ *Calculus Macacae Mulattae*

Huaihua / *Flos Sophorae*

Huainiuxi / *Radix Achyranthis Bidentatae*

Huaishanyao / *Rhizoma Dioscoreae*

Huajuhong / *Exocarpium Citri Grandis*

Huangbo / *Cortex Phellodendri*

Huangguateng / *Caulis Cucumidis Sativi*

Huangjing / *Rhizoma Polygonati*

Huanglian / *Rhizoma Coptidis*

Huangqi / *Radix Astragali*

Huangqin / *Radix Scutellariae*

Huomaren / *Fructus Cannabis*

J

Jianghuang / *Rhizoma Curcumae Longae*

Jiaobinlang / *Semen Arecae Preparata*

Jicai / *Herba Capsellae*

汉防己

旱莲草

旱芹菜

黑山栀子

黑芝麻

何首乌

荷叶

红花

红枣

猴枣

槐花

怀牛膝

怀山药

化橘红

黄柏

黄瓜藤

黄精

黄连

黄芪

黄芩

火麻仁

姜黄

焦槟榔

荠菜

高血压病的中医特色疗法

Jingjie / *Herba Schizonepetae*

Jingjiesui / *Spica Schizonepetae*

Jiudahuang / *Radix et Rhizoma Rhei Preparata*

Jiuqu / *Massa Fermentata Vinum*

Jixueteng / *Caulis Spatholobi*

Juemingzi / *Semen Cassiae*

Juhong / *Exocarpium Citri Rubrum*

Juhua / *Flos Chrysanthemi*

Juluo / *Vascular Aurantii Citri Tangerinea*

K

Kudingcha / *Folium Ilicis*

L

Lianqiao / *Fructus Forsythiae*

Lianxu / *Stamen Nelumbinis*

Lianzixin / *Plumula Nelumbinis*

Lingcishi / *Magnetitum*

Lingyangfen / *Pulvis Cornu Saigae Tataricae*

Lingyangjiao / *Cornu Saigae Tataricae*

Lingzhi / *Ganoderma Lucidum seu Japonicum*

Liuhuang / *Sulfur*

Longchi / *Dens Draconis*

Longdancao / *Radix Gentianae*

Longgu / *Os Draconis*

Luobumaye / *Folium Apocyni Veneti*

Luoshiteng / *Caulis Trachelospermi*

荆芥

荆芥穗

酒大黄

酒曲

鸡血藤

决明子

橘红

菊花

橘络

苦丁茶

连翘

莲须

莲子心

灵磁石

羚羊粉

羚羊角

灵芝

硫黄

龙齿

龙胆草

龙骨

罗布麻叶

络石藤

高血压病的中医特色疗法

Lurong / *Cornu Cervi Pantotrichum*

Lü'emei / *Flos Mume*

M

Madouling / *Fructus Aristolochiae*

Maimendong / *Radix Ophiopogonis*

Malan / *Herba Kalimeridis Indicae*

Malantou / *Rhizoma Kalimeridis Indicae*

Mangxiao / *Natrii Sulfas*

Manjingzi / *Fructus Viticis*

Maren / *Semen Cannabis*

Mingtianma / *Rhizoma Gastrodiae*

Mohanlian / *Herba Ecliptae*

Mudanpi / *Cortex Moutan*

Muli / *Concha Ostreae*

Mutong / *Caulis Akebiae*

N

Nanxing / *Rhizoma Arisaematis*

Niuhuang / *Calculus Bovis*

Niuxi / *Radix Achyranthis Bidentatae*

Nüzhenzi / *Fructus Ligustri Lucidi*

P

Paofuzi / *Radix Aconiti Lateralis Preparata*

Penghaocai / *Caulis et Folium Chrysanthemi Coronarii*

Pianjianghuang / *Rhizoma Wenyujin Concisa* , sliced

Puhuang / *Pollen Typhae*

鹿茸

绿萼梅

马兜铃

麦门冬

马兰

马兰头

芒硝

蔓荆子

麻仁

明天麻

墨旱连

牡丹皮

牡蛎

木通

南星

牛黄

牛膝

女贞子

炮附子

蓬蒿菜

片姜黄

蒲黄

高血压病的中医特色疗法

Q

Qingbanxia / *Rhizoma Pinelliae*

Qingmuxiang / *Radix Aristolochiae*

Qingpi / *Pericarpium Citri Reticulatae Viride*

Qinpi / *Cortex Fraxini*

Quangualou / *Fructus Trichosanthis*

Quanxie / *Scorpio*

Quanxiewei / *Cauda Scorpio*

R

Roucongrong / *Herba Cistanches*

Rougui / *Cortex Cinnamomi*

Rouguixin / *Lignum Cinnamomi*

Ruxiang / *Olibanum*

S

Sangbaipi / *Cortex Mori*

Sangjisheng / *Herba Taxilli*

Sangpiaoxiao / *Oötheca Mantidis*

Sangshen / *Fructus Mori*

Sangshenzi / *Fructus Mori*

Sangshugen / *Radix Mori*

Sangshupi / *Cortex Mori*

Sangzhi / *Ramulus Mori*

Sanqi / *Radix Notoginseng*

Shanlucha / *Folium Ilicis Hainanensis*

Shanyao / *Rhizoma Dioscoreae*

索　引

清半夏

青木香

青皮

秦皮

全瓜蒌

全蝎

全蝎尾

肉苁蓉

肉桂

肉桂心

乳香

桑白皮

桑寄生

桑螵蛸

桑椹

桑椹子

桑树根

桑树皮

桑枝

三七

山绿茶

山药

Shanzhuyu / *Fructus Corni*

Shanzha / *Fructus Crataegi*

Shanzhizi / *Fructus Gardeniae*

Shayuanzi / *Semen Astragali Complanati*

Shengbaishao / *Radix Paeoniae Alba*

Shengdaizheshi / *Haematitum*

Shengdihuang / *Radix Rehmanniae*

Shenghuaimi / *Flos Sophorae*

Shenghuangqi / *Radix Astragali*

Shenglonggu / *Os Draconis*

Shengmuli / *Concha Ostreae*

Shengshanzharou / *Fructus Crataegi*

Shengshanzhizi / *Fructus Gardeniae*

Shengshigao / *Gypsum Fibrosum*

Shengshijueming / *Concha Haliotidis*

Shexiang / *Moschus*

Shichangpu / *Rhizoma Acori Tatarinowii*

Shihu / *Herba Dendrobii*

Shijueming / *Concha Haliotidis*

Shudihuang / *Radix Rehmanniae Preparata*

Shufuzi / *Radix Aconiti Lateralis Preparata*

Suanzaoren / *Semen Ziziphi Spinosae*

T

Taizishen / *Radix Pseudostellariae*

Tanxiang / *Lignum Santali Albi*

山茱萸

山楂

山栀子

沙苑子

生白芍

生代赭石

生地黄

生槐米

生黄芪

生龙骨

生牡蛎

生山楂肉

生山栀子

生石膏

生石决明

麝香

石菖蒲

石斛

石决明

熟地黄

熟附子

酸枣仁

太子参

檀香

Taoren / *Semen Persicae*

Tianmendong / *Radix Asparagi*

Tianma / *Rhizoma Gastrodiae*

Tianqipian / *Radix Notoginseng*, *sliced*

Tianxianteng / *Herba Aristolochiae*

Tianzhuhuang / *Concretio Silicea Bambusae*

W

Wancansha / *Feculae Bombycis*

Wugong / *Scolopendra*

Wulingzhi / *Faeces Trogopterori*

Wuweizi / *Fructus Schisandrae*

Wuzhualong / *Radix seu Folium Ipomoeae Cairicae*

Wuzhuyu / *Fructus Evodiae*

X

Xiakucao / *Spica Prunellae*

Xiangfu / *Rhizoma Cyperi*

Xianlingpi / *Herba Epimedii*

Xianmao / *Rhizoma Curculiginis*

Xianshuqucao / *Herba Gnaphalii Affinis*, *fresh*

Xiaoji / *Herba Cirsii*

Xiaojicao / *Herba Cirsii*

Xiongdan / *Fel Ursi*

Xixiancao / *Herba Siegesbeckiae*

Xixin / *Herba Asari*

Xuanfuhua / *Flos Inulae*

桃仁

天门冬

天麻

田七片

天仙藤

天竺黄

晚蚕沙

蜈蚣

五灵脂

五味子

五爪龙

吴茱萸

夏枯草

香附

仙灵脾

仙茅

鲜鼠曲草

小蓟

小蓟草

熊胆

豨莶草

细辛

旋覆花

高血压病的中医特色疗法

Xuanshen / *Radix Scrophulariae*

Xuduan / *Radix Dipsaci*

Y

Yama / *Herba Lini*

Yanhusuo / *Rhizoma Corydalis*

Yejiaoteng / *Caulis et Folium Polygoni Multiflori*

Yejuhua / *Flos Chrysanthemi Indici*

Yimucao / *Herba Leonuri*

Yinchen / *Herba Artemisiae Scopariae*

Yinyanghuo / *Herba Epimedii*

Yiyiren / *Semen Coicis*

Yizhiren / *Fructus Alpiniae Oxyphyllae*

Yuanzhi / *Radix Polygalae*

Yujin / *Radix Curcumae*

Yulanhua / *Flos Magnoliae Denudatae*

Yumixu / *Stylus Zeae Maydis*

Yunfuling / *Poria*

Yuzhu / *Rhizoma Polygonati Odorati*

Z

Zexie / *Rhizoma Alismatis*

Zhechong / *Eupolyphaga seu Steleophaga*

Zhenzhumu / *Concha Margaritifera Usta*

Zhibiejia / *Carapax Trionycis Preparata*

Zhidanxing / *Rhizoma Arisaematis Preparata*

Zhifuzi / *Radix Aconiti Lateralis Preparata*

玄参

续断

亚麻

延胡索

夜交藤

野菊花

益母草

茵陈

淫羊藿

薏苡仁

益智仁

远志

郁金

玉兰花

玉米须

云茯苓

玉竹

泽泻

䗪虫

珍珠母

炙鳖甲

制胆星

制附子

高血压病的中医特色疗法

Zhigancao / *Radix Glycyrrhizae Preparata*

Zhiguiban / *Carapax et Plastrum Testudinis Preparata*

Zhiheshouwu / *Radix Polygoni Multiflori Preparata*

Zhihuangjing / *Rhizoma Polygonati Preparata*

Zhibaijiangcan / *Bombyx Batryticatus Preparata*

Zhike / *Fructus Aurantii*

Zhimu / *Rhizoma Anemarrhenae*

Zhinanxing / *Rhizoma Arisaematis Preparata*

Zhinüzhenzi / *Fructus Ligustri Lucidi Preparata*

Zhishi / *Fructus Aurantii Immaturus*

Zhizi / *Fructus Gardeniae*

Zhuli / *Succus Phyllostachydis Henonis*

Zhulibanxia / *Rhizoma Pinelliae et Succus Bambusae*

Zhuling / *Polyporus*

Zhuru / *Caulis Bambusae in Taeniam*

Zhusha / *Cinnabaris*

Ziheche / *Placenta Hominis*

Zisugeng / *Caulis Perillae*

Zisuzi / *Fructus Perillae*

索 引

炙甘草

炙龟版

制何首乌

制黄精

炙白僵蚕

枳壳

知母

制南星

炙女贞子

枳实

栀子

竹沥

竹沥半夏

猪苓

竹茹

朱砂

紫河车

紫苏梗

紫苏子

高血压病的中医特色疗法

An English-Chinese Guide to Clinical Treatment of Common Diseases

Typical TCM Therapy for Viral Hepatitis

Typical TCM Therapy for Primary Glomerulonephritis

Typical TCM Therapy for Chronic Gastritis

Typical TCM Therapy for Lung Cancer

Typical TCM Therapy for Bronchial Asthma

Typical TCM Therapy for Diabetes

Typical TCM Therapy for Primary Hypertension

Typical TCM Therapy for Rheumatoid Arthritis

Typical TCM Therapy for Cervical Spondylosis

Typical TCM Therapy for Cholelithiasis

（英汉对照）常见病临证要览

病毒性肝炎的中医特色疗法

原发性肾小球肾炎的中医特色疗法

慢性胃炎的中医特色疗法

肺癌的中医特色疗法

支气管哮喘的中医特色疗法

糖尿病的中医特色疗法

高血压病的中医特色疗法

类风湿关节炎的中医特色疗法

颈椎病的中医特色疗法

胆石症的中医特色疗法